Acid Reflux

Everything You Need To Know To Prepare For Live with and Treat GERD And Heartburn

Ethan D. Anderson

Xspurts.com

A New Zealand Designed Product

Other Versions Available

Why limit yourself to just one format?

This book is now available in physical, digital, and audiobook options.

Choose the way you love to read and dive into the story today. You won't regret it!

Digital ISBN: 9781776969852
Physical ISBN: 9781776969845
Audio ISBN:

To obtain a different format of this book at a discounted price, please get in touch with us at:

http://isbn.xspurts.com/

Contents

Have Questions / Comments?

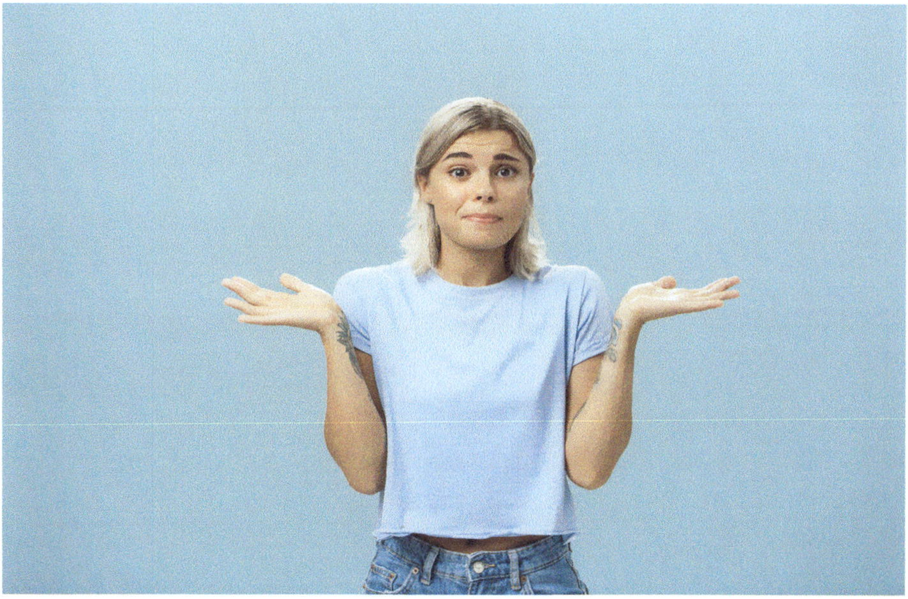

This book was designed to cover as much information as possible, but I know I have probably missed something, or some new amazing discovery has just come out.

If you notice something missing or have a question that I failed to answer, please get in touch and let me know. If I can, I will email you an answer and also update the book so others can also benefit from it.

Thanks For Being Awesome :)

Submit Your Questions / Comments At:

https://questions.xspurts.com

Get Free Stuff

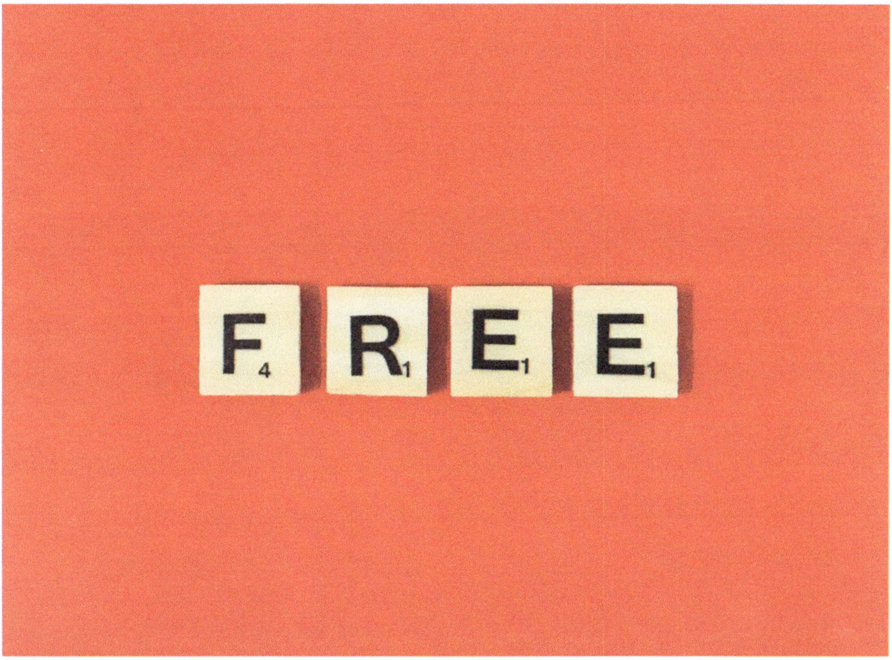

We love writing and have produced a huge number of books.

For being one of our amazing readers, we would love to offer you more books we have created, 100% free.

To claim this limited time special offer, simply go to the site below and enter your name and email address.

You will then receive loads (as we love our readers so much :) of our great books, content and audio direct to your email account, 100% free!

Get Loads of FREE Stuff at:

https://free.xspurts.com

Chapter One

Introduction

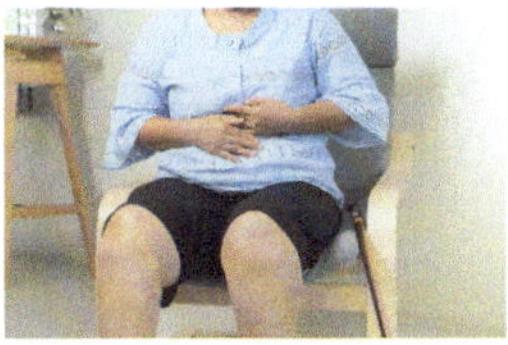

Acid Reflux: Everything You Need To Know To Prepare For Live with and Treat GERD And Heartburn is the perfect book for those who suffer from Acid Reflux and want to learn everything they need to know about the condition.

This book covers a wide range of topics such as the causes of Acid Reflux, the symptoms, the treatments and how to live with the condition.The book is full of useful information, valuable tips and advice and has been created in an easy to read and understand format.

If you suffer from Acid Reflux, or know someone who does, then this book is a must-read. It will help you to understand the condition and will provide you with the knowledge you need to manage it effectively.

Chapter Two

What is Acid Reflux?

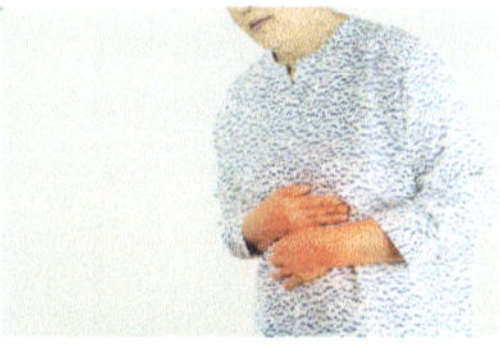

Acid reflux, also known as gastroesophageal reflux (GER), is a common digestive disorder that occurs when stomach acid and sometimes bile flows back into the esophagus. The esophagus is the tube that connects the mouth to the stomach. Normally, a ring of muscle called the lower esophageal sphincter (LES) prevents stomach acid from entering the esophagus. But when the LES relaxes or weakens, acid can leak into the esophagus, causing a burning sensation in the chest and throat.

Symptoms of acid reflux can vary, but common signs and symptoms include:

Heartburn, a burning sensation in the chest that can radiate to the neck, throat, or jaw

Regurgitation, a sour or bitter taste in the mouth or throat

Difficulty swallowing

Coughing or wheezing

Chest pain

Acid reflux can be an occasional or chronic condition. Occasional acid reflux is generally not a cause for concern, but chronic acid reflux can lead to more serious complications, such as esophagitis (inflammation of the esophagus), Barrett's esophagus (a precancerous condition), and esophageal cancer.

There are several factors that can contribute to the development of acid reflux, including:

Hiatal hernia: a condition in which part of the stomach protrudes through the diaphragm into the chest cavity, causing the LES to malfunction.

Obesity: Excess body weight can increase pressure on the stomach, causing acid to flow back into the esophagus.

Pregnancy: Hormonal changes and increased pressure on the abdomen during pregnancy can cause acid reflux.

Smoking: Smoking weakens the LES and increases acid production in the stomach.

Certain foods and beverages: Certain foods and drinks can trigger acid reflux, including spicy foods, fatty foods, citrus fruits, tomatoes, chocolate, caffeine, and alcohol.

Treatment for acid reflux generally involves lifestyle modifications and medication. Lifestyle modifications may include:

Avoiding trigger foods and beverages

Eating smaller, more frequent meals

Avoiding lying down for at least three hours after eating

Elevating the head of the bed

Losing weight if necessary

Quitting smoking

Medications for acid reflux include:

Antacids: Over-the-counter antacids, such as Tums and Maalox, can neutralize stomach acid.

H2 blockers: Prescription or over-the-counter medications, such as famotidine (Pepcid) and ranitidine (Zantac), can reduce the amount of acid produced by the stomach.

Proton pump inhibitors (PPIs): Prescription or over-the-counter medications, such as omeprazole (Prilosec) and lansoprazole (Prevacid), can block acid production in the stomach.

In some cases, surgery may be necessary to treat acid reflux that does not respond to medication or lifestyle changes.

If you experience symptoms of acid reflux, it's important to speak with your healthcare provider to determine the best course of treatment. With the right approach, acid reflux can be effectively managed, allowing you to enjoy a healthy, comfortable digestive system.

Chapter Three

The different types of Acid Reflux

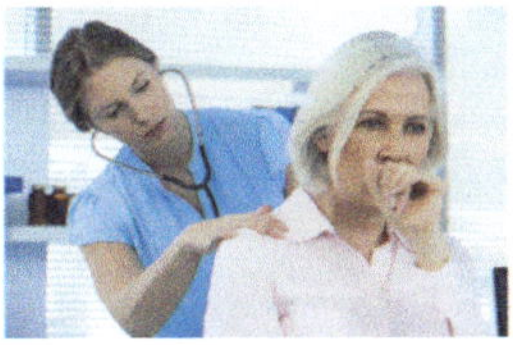

Acid reflux, also known as gastroesophageal reflux (GER), can manifest in different ways depending on the severity of the condition and the specific symptoms experienced by the individual. There are several types of acid reflux, including:

Occasional acid reflux: This is the most common type of acid reflux and is experienced by most people at some point in their lives. Occasional acid reflux typically occurs when the lower esophageal sphincter (LES) relaxes or weakens, allowing stomach acid to flow back into the esophagus. Occasional acid reflux may be triggered by certain foods or beverages, such as spicy or fatty foods, caffeine, or alcohol.

Gastroesophageal reflux disease (GERD): GERD is a chronic condition in which acid reflux occurs at least twice a week, leading to persistent symptoms such as heartburn, regurgitation, and difficulty swallowing. GERD can be caused by a variety of factors, including a weak LES, a hiatal hernia, obesity, or pregnancy.

Silent reflux: Silent reflux, also known as laryngopharyngeal reflux (LPR), occurs when stomach acid flows back into the throat and voice box, leading to symptoms such as hoarseness, chronic cough, and difficulty swallowing.

Unlike traditional acid reflux, silent reflux may not cause heartburn or other digestive symptoms, making it difficult to diagnose.

Reflux esophagitis: Reflux esophagitis is a complication of GERD in which the lining of the esophagus becomes inflamed and irritated due to prolonged exposure to stomach acid. Symptoms of reflux esophagitis may include difficulty swallowing, chest pain, and persistent heartburn.

Barrett's esophagus: Barrett's esophagus is a rare but serious complication of GERD in which the cells in the lining of the esophagus become abnormal and increase the risk of esophageal cancer. Barrett's esophagus may be asymptomatic or may cause symptoms such as difficulty swallowing or chest pain.

The treatment for acid reflux depends on the type and severity of the condition. Occasional acid reflux can often be managed with lifestyle modifications and over-the-counter antacids, while more severe or chronic cases may require prescription medications or surgery. If you suspect that you may have acid reflux, it's important to speak with your healthcare provider to determine the best course of treatment.

Chapter Four

Occasional acid reflux

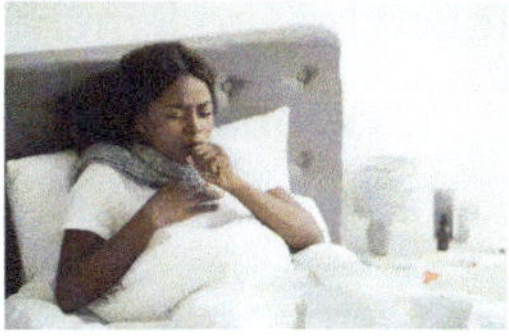

Occasional acid reflux is the most common type of acid reflux and is experienced by most people at some point in their lives. It occurs when the lower esophageal sphincter (LES) relaxes or weakens, allowing stomach acid to flow back into the esophagus.

Symptoms of occasional acid reflux may include heartburn, a burning sensation in the chest or throat, and a sour or bitter taste in the mouth. These symptoms are often triggered by certain foods or beverages, such as spicy or fatty foods, caffeine, or alcohol.

Occasional acid reflux can typically be managed with lifestyle modifications and over-the-counter antacids. Here are some tips that may help reduce the frequency and severity of occasional acid reflux:

Avoid trigger foods: If you notice that certain foods or beverages trigger your acid reflux symptoms, try to avoid them as much as possible. Common trigger foods include spicy or fatty foods, chocolate, caffeine, and alcohol.

Eat smaller meals: Eating smaller, more frequent meals throughout the day can help reduce the amount of acid produced in the stomach, which may reduce the risk of acid reflux.

Don't lie down after eating: Wait at least 3 hours after eating before lying down or going to bed. This can help prevent stomach acid from flowing back into the esophagus.

Elevate the head of your bed: Raising the head of your bed by 6 to 8 inches can help prevent stomach acid from flowing back into the esophagus while you sleep.

Quit smoking: Smoking can weaken the LES and increase the risk of acid reflux.

Manage stress: Stress can trigger or worsen acid reflux symptoms, so finding ways to manage stress, such as exercise, meditation, or deep breathing, may be helpful.

If lifestyle modifications and over-the-counter antacids do not provide relief from occasional acid reflux, your healthcare provider may recommend prescription medications or further testing to determine the underlying cause of your symptoms. It's important to speak with your healthcare provider if you experience frequent or severe acid reflux symptoms to determine the best course of treatment.

Chapter Five

Silent reflux / Laryngopharyngeal Reflux (LPR)

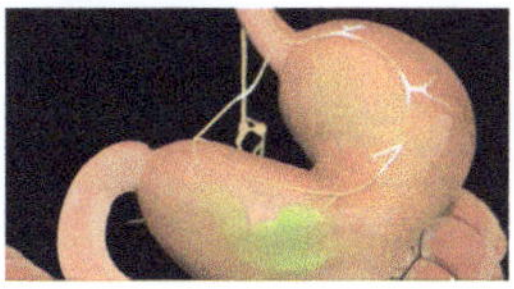

Silent reflux, also known as laryngopharyngeal reflux (LPR), is a type of acid reflux that affects the throat and voice box. Unlike traditional acid reflux, which is typically characterized by heartburn and a burning sensation in the chest, silent reflux may not cause any noticeable symptoms in the esophagus. Instead, the acid refluxes up into the throat, which can lead to irritation and inflammation.

Symptoms of silent reflux may include:

Hoarseness or a change in the voice

Chronic cough

Throat clearing

Postnasal drip

Difficulty swallowing

Sore throat

Bad breath

Ear pain

Silent reflux is often triggered by the same factors that can trigger traditional acid reflux, such as certain foods, beverages, and lifestyle habits. However, there are some additional factors that may increase the risk of developing silent reflux, such as:

Obesity

Pregnancy

Smoking

Hiatal hernia

Asthma

Treatment for silent reflux typically involves lifestyle modifications and medications to reduce the amount of acid produced in the stomach. Here are some tips that may help reduce the frequency and severity of silent reflux:

Avoid trigger foods: Certain foods and beverages can trigger silent reflux, so try to avoid them as much as possible. Common trigger foods include spicy or fatty foods, caffeine, chocolate, and alcohol.

Eat smaller meals: Eating smaller, more frequent meals throughout the day can help reduce the amount of acid produced in the stomach, which may reduce the risk of silent reflux.

Don't lie down after eating: Wait at least 3 hours after eating before lying down or going to bed. This can help prevent stomach acid from flowing back into the esophagus.

Elevate the head of your bed: Raising the head of your bed by 6 to 8 inches can help prevent stomach acid from flowing back into the esophagus while you sleep.

Quit smoking: Smoking can weaken the lower esophageal sphincter (LES) and increase the risk of silent reflux.

Manage stress: Stress can trigger or worsen silent reflux symptoms, so finding ways to manage stress, such as exercise, meditation, or deep breathing, may be helpful.

In addition to these lifestyle modifications, your healthcare provider may recommend medications to reduce the amount of acid produced in the stomach, such as proton pump inhibitors (PPIs) or H2 blockers. In some cases, your healthcare provider may recommend surgery to strengthen the LES and prevent stomach acid from flowing back into the esophagus.

If you experience frequent or severe symptoms of silent reflux, it's important to speak with your healthcare provider to determine the best course of treatment for your individual needs.

Chapter Six

Gerd / Gastroesophageal Reflux

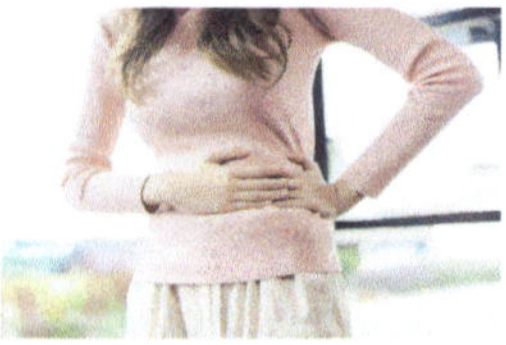

Gastroesophageal reflux disease (GERD) is a chronic digestive disorder that occurs when stomach acid or bile flows back into the esophagus, causing irritation and inflammation. GERD is a more severe and chronic form of acid reflux, with symptoms that can have a significant impact on a person's quality of life.

Symptoms of GERD may include:

Heartburn, a burning sensation in the chest that may occur after eating or lying down

Regurgitation, the sensation of acid flowing back into the mouth or throat

Nausea

Difficulty swallowing

Chest pain

Chronic cough

Hoarseness or sore throat

Asthma

GERD is often caused by a malfunctioning lower esophageal sphincter (LES), the ring of muscle that separates the esophagus from the stomach. When the LES doesn't close properly, stomach acid can flow back into the esophagus, causing irritation and inflammation.

There are several factors that can increase the risk of developing GERD, including:

Obesity

Pregnancy

Hiatal hernia

Smoking

Alcohol consumption

Certain medications, such as antihistamines, calcium channel blockers, and nitrates

Treatment for GERD typically involves lifestyle modifications and medications to reduce the amount of acid produced in the stomach. Here are some tips that may help reduce the frequency and severity of GERD:

Avoid trigger foods: Certain foods and beverages can trigger GERD, so try to avoid them as much as possible. Common trigger foods include spicy or fatty foods, caffeine, chocolate, and alcohol.

Eat smaller meals: Eating smaller, more frequent meals throughout the day can help reduce the amount of acid produced in the stomach, which may reduce the risk of GERD.

Don't lie down after eating: Wait at least 3 hours after eating before lying down or going to bed. This can help prevent stomach acid from flowing back into the esophagus.

Elevate the head of your bed: Raising the head of your bed by 6 to 8 inches can help prevent stomach acid from flowing back into the esophagus while you sleep.

Quit smoking: Smoking can weaken the lower esophageal sphincter (LES) and increase the risk of GERD.

Manage stress: Stress can trigger or worsen GERD symptoms, so finding ways to manage stress, such as exercise, meditation, or deep breathing, may be helpful.

In addition to these lifestyle modifications, your healthcare provider may recommend medications to reduce the amount of acid produced in the stomach, such as proton pump inhibitors (PPIs) or H2 blockers. In some cases, your healthcare provider may recommend surgery to strengthen the LES and prevent stomach acid from flowing back into the esophagus.

If you experience frequent or severe symptoms of GERD, it's important to speak with your healthcare provider to determine the best course of treatment for your individual needs. Untreated GERD can lead to complications such as esophagitis, esophageal ulcers, and Barrett's esophagus, a condition that increases the risk of developing esophageal cancer.

Chapter Seven

Reflux esophagitis

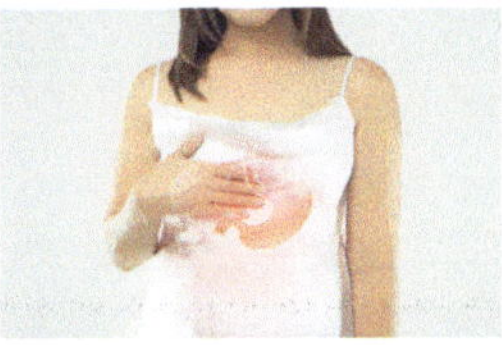

Reflux esophagitis is a type of gastroesophageal reflux disease (GERD) that is caused by inflammation and irritation of the lining of the esophagus due to chronic acid exposure. It is a more severe form of GERD and can lead to complications such as ulcers, bleeding, and strictures (narrowing of the esophagus).

GERD occurs when stomach acid and other contents of the digestive system flow back up into the esophagus, causing symptoms such as heartburn, regurgitation, and difficulty swallowing. Reflux esophagitis is characterized by the presence of inflammation and irritation in the lining of the esophagus, which can be seen on an endoscopy.

Symptoms of reflux esophagitis include heartburn, chest pain, difficulty swallowing, and nausea. In severe cases, patients may experience vomiting, bleeding, or unintentional weight loss. It is important to see a doctor if you experience persistent symptoms of reflux esophagitis, as it can lead to more serious complications over time.

Treatment for reflux esophagitis involves reducing acid production in the stomach, improving the function of the lower esophageal sphincter (the muscle that separates the esophagus from the stomach), and protecting the lining of the esophagus from further damage. This may involve lifestyle changes such as weight loss, avoiding trigger foods, and elevating the head of the bed while sleeping. Medications such as proton pump inhibitors (PPIs) and H2 blockers can also be used to reduce acid production.

In some cases, surgical intervention may be necessary to repair the lower esophageal sphincter or to remove damaged tissue from the esophagus. Your doctor can help determine the most appropriate treatment plan for your individual case of reflux esophagitis.

Chapter Eight

Barrett's esophagus

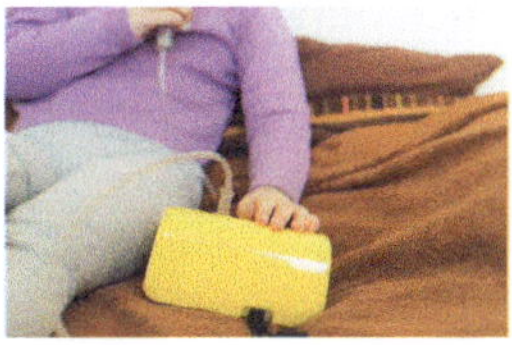

Barrett's esophagus is a condition in which the lining of the esophagus is replaced with tissue that is similar to the lining of the intestine. It is a complication of gastroesophageal reflux disease (GERD) and is associated with an increased risk of developing esophageal cancer.

GERD occurs when stomach acid and other contents of the digestive system flow back up into the esophagus, causing symptoms such as heartburn, regurgitation, and difficulty swallowing. Over time, the chronic exposure to acid can cause changes in the lining of the esophagus. In some cases, this can lead to the development of Barrett's esophagus.

Barrett's esophagus often does not cause any symptoms, but it can be diagnosed through an endoscopy, which is a procedure in which a flexible tube with a camera on the end is inserted into the esophagus. During the endoscopy, the doctor can take a biopsy of the tissue in the esophagus to confirm the diagnosis of Barrett's esophagus.

Because of the increased risk of esophageal cancer associated with Barrett's esophagus, patients with this condition are often monitored closely with regular endoscopies and biopsies. Treatment for Barrett's esophagus may involve medications to reduce acid production in the stomach and lifestyle changes to reduce the risk of further damage to the esophagus.

In some cases, more aggressive treatment may be necessary, such as endoscopic resection of the abnormal tissue or surgery to remove a portion of the esophagus. Your doctor can help determine the most appropriate treatment plan for your individual case of Barrett's esophagus.

It is important to seek medical attention if you experience persistent symptoms of GERD, such as heartburn or difficulty swallowing, as this can increase the risk of developing Barrett's esophagus and other complications.

Chapter Nine

Precancer or cancer

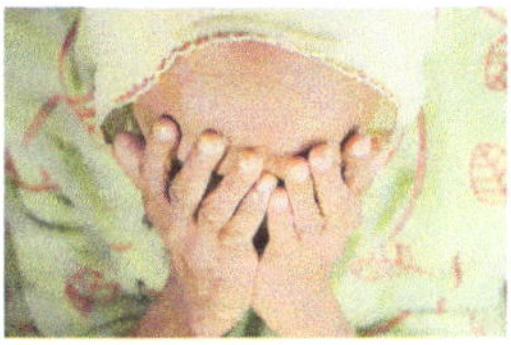

Esophageal cancer is a type of cancer that starts in the cells lining the esophagus, the muscular tube that carries food and liquids from the throat to the stomach. Chronic gastroesophageal reflux disease (GERD) is a known risk factor for developing esophageal cancer.

When stomach acid and other contents of the digestive system flow back up into the esophagus over a long period of time, it can cause chronic inflammation and irritation of the lining of the esophagus. This can lead to the development of changes in the cells of the esophagus, a condition called Barrett's esophagus, which is a precursor to esophageal cancer.

The risk of developing esophageal cancer from GERD is relatively low, but the risk increases with the duration and severity of the disease. Other factors that can increase the risk of developing esophageal cancer include smoking, heavy alcohol use, obesity, and a family history of the disease.

Symptoms of esophageal cancer may include difficulty swallowing, chest pain, weight loss, and persistent cough. However, in some cases, there may be no symptoms until the cancer has spread to other parts of the body.

Diagnosis of esophageal cancer usually involves an endoscopy, which is a procedure in which a flexible tube with a camera on the end is inserted into the esophagus. During the endoscopy, the doctor can take a biopsy of the tissue in the esophagus to confirm the diagnosis of esophageal cancer.

Treatment for esophageal cancer depends on the stage of the disease and may include surgery, radiation therapy, and chemotherapy. Early detection is key to successful treatment, so it is important to seek medical attention if you experience any persistent symptoms of GERD or other symptoms that may be related to esophageal cancer.

Prevention of esophageal cancer involves managing risk factors, such as quitting smoking, reducing alcohol consumption, and maintaining a healthy weight. Treatment of GERD may also help reduce the risk of developing esophageal cancer. If you have a family history of esophageal cancer or other risk factors, talk to your doctor about whether you may be a candidate for screening tests to detect the disease early.

Chapter Ten

Who's at risk for Acid Reflux

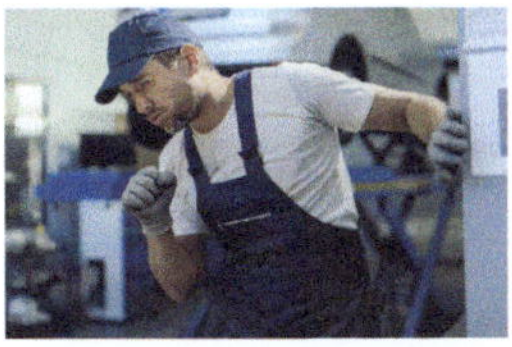

Acid reflux can affect anyone, but certain factors can increase the risk of developing the condition. Some of the common risk factors for acid reflux include:

Obesity: Excess weight can put pressure on the stomach, forcing stomach acid back up into the esophagus.

Pregnancy: The increased pressure on the stomach during pregnancy can cause acid reflux.

Hiatal hernia: A hiatal hernia is a condition in which the upper part of the stomach bulges through the diaphragm into the chest cavity. This can make it easier for stomach acid to flow back up into the esophagus.

Smoking: Smoking weakens the lower esophageal sphincter, the muscle that normally prevents stomach acid from flowing back up into the esophagus.

Certain foods and drinks: Certain foods and drinks, such as citrus fruits, tomatoes, chocolate, caffeine, and alcohol, can trigger acid reflux in some people.

Medications: Certain medications, such as aspirin and other nonsteroidal anti-inflammatory drugs (NSAIDs), can irritate the lining of the esophagus and increase the risk of acid reflux.

Stress: Stress can increase the production of stomach acid, which can trigger acid reflux.

Age: The risk of acid reflux increases with age, as the muscles that support the esophagus weaken over time.

It's important to note that while these risk factors may increase the likelihood of developing acid reflux, not everyone with these risk factors will develop the condition. If you are at risk for acid reflux, there are steps you can take to reduce your risk, such as maintaining a healthy weight, avoiding trigger foods and drinks, quitting smoking, and managing stress.

Chapter Eleven

How do you get Acid Reflux

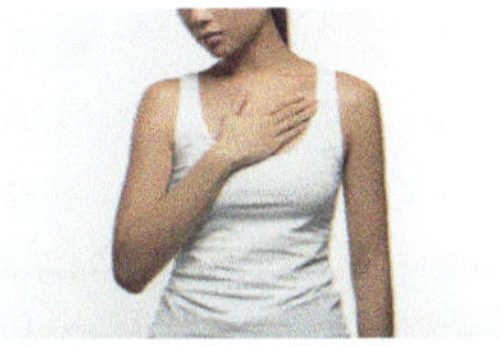

Acid reflux occurs when the muscle at the lower end of the esophagus, called the lower esophageal sphincter (LES), doesn't close properly, allowing stomach acid to flow back up into the esophagus. This can cause a burning sensation in the chest or throat, known as heartburn.

The most common cause of acid reflux is eating a large or fatty meal, which can put pressure on the LES and cause it to relax. Other factors that can contribute to acid reflux include:

Eating certain trigger foods: Certain foods, such as citrus fruits, tomatoes, chocolate, caffeine, and alcohol, can trigger acid reflux in some people.

Overeating: Eating large meals or overeating can put pressure on the LES, allowing stomach acid to flow back up into the esophagus.

Eating before bedtime: Eating a large meal or snacking before bedtime can increase the likelihood of acid reflux, as lying down can make it easier for stomach acid to flow back up into the esophagus.

Hiatal hernia: A hiatal hernia is a condition in which the upper part of the stomach bulges through the diaphragm into the chest cavity. This can make it easier for stomach acid to flow back up into the esophagus.

Smoking: Smoking weakens the LES, making it easier for stomach acid to flow back up into the esophagus.

Medications: Certain medications, such as aspirin and other nonsteroidal anti-inflammatory drugs (NSAIDs), can irritate the lining of the esophagus and increase the risk of acid reflux.

It's important to note that occasional acid reflux is common and usually not a cause for concern. However, if you experience frequent or severe acid reflux, you should talk to your doctor, as this can be a sign of a more serious condition such as gastroesophageal reflux disease (GERD) or Barrett's esophagus.

Chapter Twelve

What are the symptoms of Acid Reflux

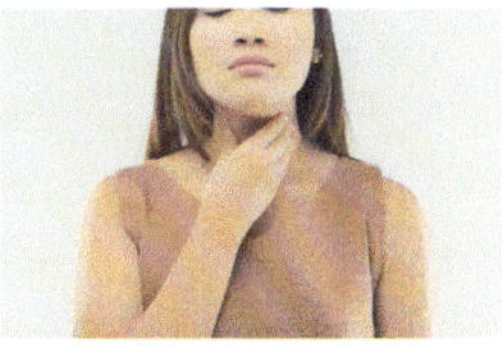

The most common symptom of acid reflux is heartburn, which is a burning sensation in the chest or throat that occurs after eating or lying down. Other symptoms of acid reflux can include:

Regurgitation: A sour or bitter taste in the back of the throat, or the feeling that food or liquid is coming back up into the mouth.

Nausea: Some people with acid reflux may experience nausea or even vomiting.

Difficulty swallowing: Acid reflux can cause the muscles in the esophagus to spasm, making it difficult to swallow.

Chest pain: Chest pain that may be mistaken for a heart attack is a less common symptom of acid reflux.

Sore throat or hoarseness: Stomach acid can irritate the lining of the throat, leading to a sore throat or hoarseness.

Chronic cough: A cough that lasts for several weeks or longer may be a sign of acid reflux.

Symptoms of acid reflux may be worse at night, when lying down, or after eating a large or fatty meal. In some cases, acid reflux can lead to complications such as esophagitis, a condition in which the lining of the esophagus becomes inflamed, or Barrett's esophagus, a precancerous condition that can lead to esophageal cancer. If you experience frequent or severe acid reflux symptoms, it's important to talk to your doctor.

Chapter Thirteen

What causes Acid Reflux?

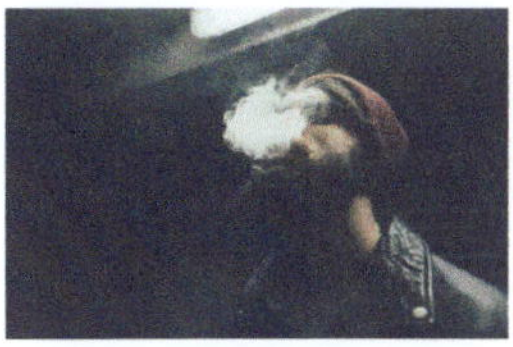

Acid reflux is caused by a malfunction of the lower esophageal sphincter (LES), which is the muscle that separates the stomach from the esophagus. Normally, the LES opens to allow food and liquids to pass into the stomach, and then closes to prevent stomach acid from flowing back into the esophagus. However, in some people, the LES does not function properly and allows acid to escape from the stomach into the esophagus. This is known as gastroesophageal reflux (GER) and is a normal occurrence in most people.

When GER occurs frequently, it is known as gastroesophageal reflux disease (GERD), which can cause damage to the lining of the esophagus. The exact cause of GERD is not fully understood, but there are several factors that can contribute to its development, including:

Hiatal hernia: This is a condition in which the upper part of the stomach protrudes through the diaphragm into the chest cavity, which can make it easier for stomach acid to flow back into the esophagus.

Obesity: Excess body weight can put pressure on the stomach, causing stomach acid to flow back into the esophagus.

Pregnancy: Hormonal changes during pregnancy can relax the LES, making it easier for stomach acid to flow back into the esophagus.

Smoking: Smoking can weaken the LES and increase acid production in the stomach.

Certain foods and drinks: Certain foods and drinks, such as citrus fruits, tomatoes, chocolate, coffee, and alcohol, can relax the LES and trigger acid reflux.

Medications: Some medications, such as aspirin, ibuprofen, and certain blood pressure medications, can irritate the lining of the esophagus and trigger acid reflux.

Stress: Stress can cause the body to produce more stomach acid, which can increase the risk of acid reflux.

Age: The risk of acid reflux increases with age, as the muscles that support the LES tend to weaken over time.

In some cases, acid reflux may be a symptom of a more serious condition, such as a peptic ulcer, esophageal stricture, or esophageal cancer. If you experience frequent or severe acid reflux, it's important to talk to your doctor to rule out any underlying medical conditions.

Chapter Fourteen

How can Acid Reflux be prevented?

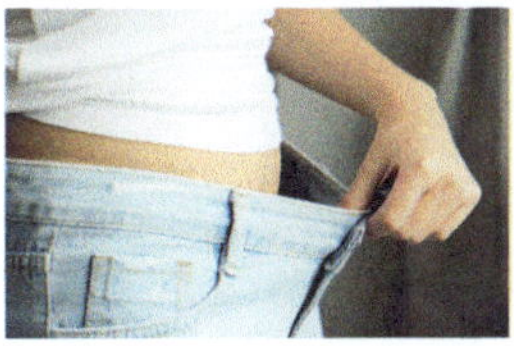

Acid reflux, also known as gastroesophageal reflux disease (GERD), is a condition that affects millions of people around the world. Although it can be uncomfortable and disruptive to daily life, there are several ways to prevent acid reflux.

Here are some tips to help prevent acid reflux:

Maintain a healthy weight: Being overweight or obese increases the risk of developing acid reflux. Extra weight around the waist puts pressure on the stomach and can cause stomach acid to back up into the esophagus. Losing weight and maintaining a healthy weight can help reduce the symptoms of acid reflux.

Avoid trigger foods: Certain foods and drinks can trigger acid reflux symptoms. Common trigger foods include fried or fatty foods, chocolate, caffeine, alcohol, citrus fruits and juices, spicy foods, and tomato-based foods. It's important to keep track of what foods trigger your symptoms and avoid them.

Eat smaller, more frequent meals: Large meals can increase pressure on the stomach and lead to acid reflux. Instead of three large meals, try eating five or six smaller meals throughout the day. This will help keep the stomach from becoming too full and prevent acid reflux.

Don't lie down after eating: Wait at least two to three hours after eating before lying down or going to bed. This allows the stomach to empty and reduces the risk of acid reflux.

Elevate the head of your bed: Elevating the head of your bed by six to eight inches can help prevent acid reflux at night. This can be done by placing blocks under the legs at the head of the bed or by using a wedge-shaped pillow.

Quit smoking: Smoking can contribute to acid reflux by relaxing the muscles that keep stomach acid in the stomach. If you smoke, quitting can help reduce the symptoms of acid reflux.

Manage stress: Stress and anxiety can trigger acid reflux symptoms. Finding ways to manage stress, such as exercise, meditation, or talking with a therapist, can help reduce symptoms.

In conclusion, preventing acid reflux involves maintaining a healthy weight, avoiding trigger foods, eating smaller, more frequent meals, not lying down after eating, elevating the head of your bed, quitting smoking, and managing stress. These lifestyle changes can be effective in reducing the symptoms of acid reflux and improving quality of life.

Chapter Fifteen

How is Acid Reflux diagnosed?

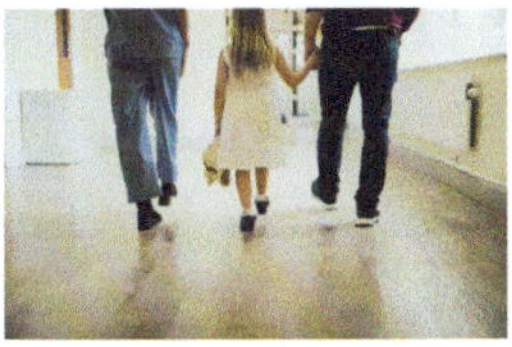

Acid reflux, or gastroesophageal reflux disease (GERD), can be diagnosed by a doctor based on your symptoms and medical history, as well as through various tests.

The first step in diagnosing acid reflux is a physical exam and a review of your symptoms. Your doctor will ask about the frequency and severity of your symptoms, such as heartburn, chest pain, difficulty swallowing, and regurgitation. They will also ask about any other medical conditions you may have and medications you are taking.

In some cases, your doctor may recommend certain tests to confirm the diagnosis of acid reflux. One test that is commonly used is an upper endoscopy, also called an esophagogastroduodenoscopy (EGD). This test involves passing a flexible tube with a camera down your throat to examine the inside of your esophagus and stomach. During this test, your doctor may take a tissue sample (biopsy) to check for inflammation or signs of other conditions, such as Barrett's esophagus.

Another test that may be used is an esophageal pH test. This test involves placing a small tube with a sensor down your esophagus to measure the acidity of the esophagus. This can help your doctor determine if you have acid reflux and how severe it is.

In some cases, imaging tests such as a barium swallow or an upper GI series may be recommended. These tests involve drinking a special liquid that can be seen on X-rays as it travels through your esophagus and stomach. This can help your doctor identify any structural abnormalities or problems with the function of your esophagus.

If you have symptoms of acid reflux, it is important to see a doctor for an accurate diagnosis and appropriate treatment. Untreated acid reflux can lead to complications such as esophagitis, Barrett's esophagus, and esophageal cancer.

Chapter Sixteen

How do you treat Acid Reflux?

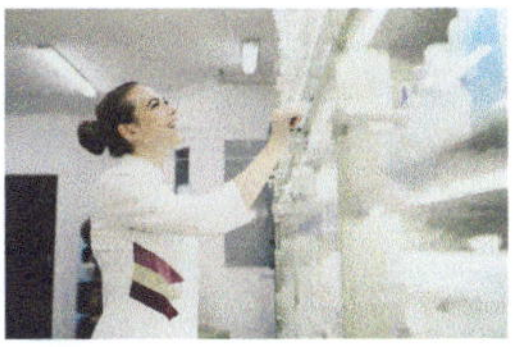

Acid reflux is a common condition that affects millions of people around the world. It can cause uncomfortable symptoms like heartburn, regurgitation, and a sour or bitter taste in the mouth. Fortunately, there are several treatment options available to help manage acid reflux.

One of the first steps in treating acid reflux is to make changes to your lifestyle and diet. For example, avoiding foods that trigger your symptoms, eating smaller meals more frequently, and avoiding eating before bedtime can help reduce symptoms. Losing weight if you are overweight can also help.

Over-the-counter medications can be effective for treating mild cases of acid reflux. Antacids like Tums, Rolaids, and Maalox can help neutralize stomach acid, while H2 blockers like Pepcid, Zantac, and Tagamet can reduce the amount of acid your stomach produces. Proton pump inhibitors (PPIs) like Nexium, Prilosec, and Prevacid are also available over the counter and can help reduce the amount of acid your stomach produces.

For more severe cases of acid reflux, prescription medications may be necessary. These can include stronger doses of H2 blockers or PPIs, as well as prokinetic agents that help your stomach empty more quickly. In some cases, surgery may be necessary to correct a hiatal hernia or to strengthen the lower esophageal sphincter.

It's important to work closely with your doctor to find the right treatment for your individual needs. In some cases, a combination of lifestyle changes and medication may be necessary to effectively manage acid reflux. With proper treatment, most people with acid reflux are able to find relief from their symptoms and enjoy a better quality of life.

Chapter Seventeen

Alternative treatments for Acid Reflux

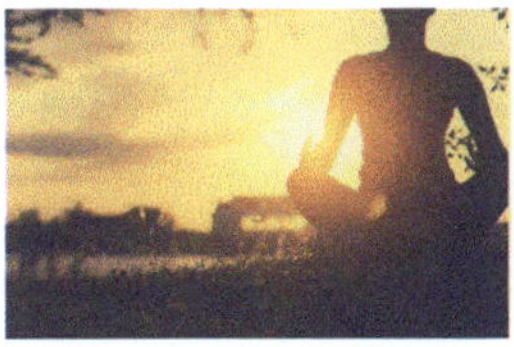

In addition to traditional medical treatments, there are also alternative approaches that some people use to manage their acid reflux symptoms. These approaches may be used in conjunction with traditional treatments or on their own. Here are a few examples of alternative treatments for acid reflux:

Herbal remedies: Some people use herbs like ginger, chamomile, and licorice root to help manage their acid reflux symptoms. These herbs can be taken in supplement form or made into teas. However, it's important to talk to your doctor before taking any herbal supplements, as they can interact with other medications.

Probiotics: Probiotics are beneficial bacteria that live in your gut and can help promote digestive health. Some studies suggest that taking probiotic supplements or eating foods that are high in probiotics, like yogurt, sauerkraut, and kimchi, can help improve acid reflux symptoms.

Acupuncture: Acupuncture is a traditional Chinese medicine practice that involves inserting thin needles into specific points on the body. Some people find that acupuncture can help relieve their acid reflux symptoms by reducing inflammation and promoting relaxation.

Mind-body techniques: Stress and anxiety can make acid reflux symptoms worse, so some people find that mind-body techniques like yoga, meditation, and deep breathing can help reduce their symptoms. These techniques can help promote relaxation and reduce stress, which can in turn help alleviate acid reflux symptoms.

Dietary changes: Making changes to your diet can also help alleviate acid reflux symptoms. Some people find that avoiding trigger foods like caffeine, alcohol, spicy foods, and citrus fruits can help reduce their symptoms. Eating smaller, more frequent meals and avoiding eating before bedtime can also be helpful.

It's important to keep in mind that not all alternative treatments are backed by scientific research, and some may not be safe for everyone. Talk to your doctor before trying any alternative treatments for acid reflux, and always follow their advice on how to manage your symptoms.

Chapter Eighteen

What is the prognosis for Acid Reflux

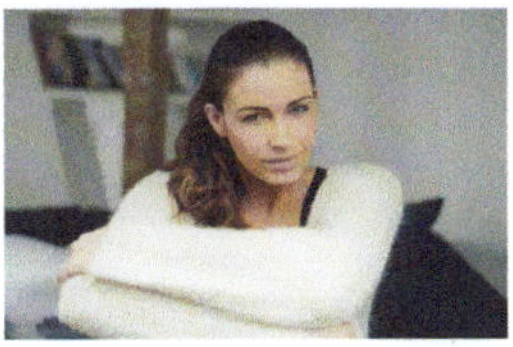

Acid reflux is a chronic condition, and the prognosis can vary depending on the severity of the symptoms and how well the condition is managed. In most cases, acid reflux can be managed with lifestyle modifications and medications, and the prognosis is good. However, if left untreated or unmanaged, acid reflux can lead to more serious complications, such as Barrett's esophagus or esophageal cancer.

With appropriate treatment, most people with acid reflux are able to control their symptoms and prevent complications. However, it is important to note that acid reflux is a chronic condition, and symptoms may continue to occur despite treatment. It is important to work closely with a healthcare provider to manage the condition and monitor for any potential complications.

In cases of Barrett's esophagus or esophageal cancer, the prognosis can be more serious. However, with early detection and treatment, the prognosis can be improved. Regular monitoring and follow-up care are essential for people with a history of acid reflux or related complications.

Chapter Nineteen

The role of diet in Acid Reflux

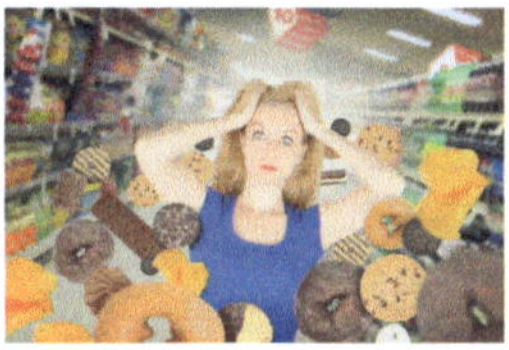

Diet plays an important role in the management of acid reflux. Certain foods and drinks can trigger symptoms, while others can help to alleviate them. While the specific triggers can vary from person to person, there are some general dietary guidelines that may be helpful for people with acid reflux.

Foods to Avoid:

High-fat foods: Foods that are high in fat can take longer to digest, which can increase the risk of acid reflux. Avoid foods like fried foods, fatty meats, and high-fat dairy products.

Spicy foods: Spicy foods can be a trigger for some people with acid reflux. Avoid foods like hot peppers, chili, and curry.

Acidic foods: Acidic foods can irritate the esophagus and trigger acid reflux symptoms. Avoid foods like citrus fruits and juices, tomatoes, and vinegar.

Carbonated beverages: Carbonated drinks can cause bloating and increase the risk of acid reflux. Avoid carbonated drinks like soda and sparkling water.

Caffeine: Caffeine can increase stomach acid production and relax the lower esophageal sphincter (LES), which can lead to acid reflux. Avoid caffeine-containing drinks like coffee, tea, and energy drinks.

Foods to Eat:

High-fiber foods: Fiber can help to reduce the risk of acid reflux by promoting regular bowel movements and preventing constipation. Good sources of fiber include fruits, vegetables, whole grains, and legumes.

Lean protein: Lean protein sources, such as chicken, fish, and tofu, can be a good option for people with acid reflux.

Non-acidic fruits: Non-acidic fruits, such as bananas, melons, and apples, can be a good option for people with acid reflux.

Vegetables: Most vegetables are low in fat and can be a good option for people with acid reflux. Avoid high-fat preparations like frying or cream-based sauces.

Alkaline water: Some people find that drinking alkaline water can help to reduce the symptoms of acid reflux. Alkaline water has a higher pH level than tap water, which can help to neutralize stomach acid.

In addition to making dietary changes, it is important to eat smaller, more frequent meals and to avoid eating before bed. Lying down after eating can increase the risk of acid reflux, so it is recommended to wait at least two hours before lying down after eating. It is also important to maintain a healthy weight, as excess weight can increase the risk of acid reflux.

Chapter Twenty

The role of stress in Acid Reflux

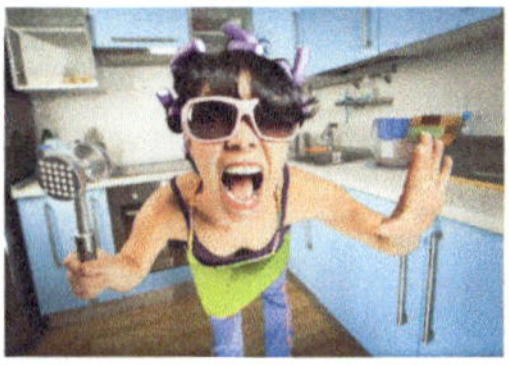

Acid reflux is a condition where the stomach acid flows back into the esophagus, causing discomfort and irritation. While diet and lifestyle choices can be contributing factors, stress can also play a role in the development and exacerbation of acid reflux.

Stress can affect the digestive system in a number of ways. When we experience stress, our bodies go into fight or flight mode, which can lead to a decrease in blood flow to the digestive system. This can cause the muscles in the digestive tract to tense up, slowing down the digestive process and leading to a buildup of acid.

Stress can also lead to the overproduction of stomach acid, as well as the relaxation of the lower esophageal sphincter, which is the muscle that controls the flow of food and acid from the esophagus to the stomach. When this muscle relaxes, it can allow stomach acid to flow back into the esophagus, causing acid reflux.

In addition to these physical effects, stress can also have a psychological impact that can worsen acid reflux symptoms. For example, stress can cause people to engage in unhealthy habits such as smoking or overeating, which can contribute to acid reflux. Stress can also lead to a lack of sleep, which can further exacerbate acid reflux symptoms.

Managing stress is an important aspect of managing acid reflux. Techniques such as meditation, deep breathing, and yoga can help to reduce stress and promote relaxation. Exercise is also a great way to relieve stress and promote a healthy digestive system. Additionally, it's important to identify and address the underlying causes of stress in order to prevent it from affecting your health.

It's also important to recognize that stress can be a trigger for acid reflux, but it is not the sole cause of the condition. Other factors such as diet, obesity, and certain medications can also contribute to the development and exacerbation of acid reflux. Therefore, it's important to work with a healthcare provider to develop a comprehensive treatment plan that takes into account all of the factors that may be contributing to your acid reflux symptoms.36

Chapter Twenty-One

What are the risks and complications associated with Acid Reflux?

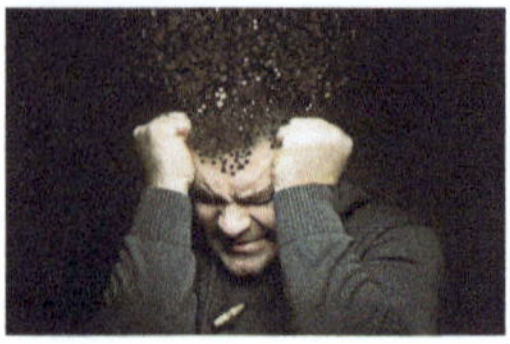

Acid reflux, also known as gastroesophageal reflux disease (GERD), is a common digestive disorder that affects many people. While it is typically not a serious condition, if left untreated, it can lead to a range of risks and complications.

One of the most common risks associated with acid reflux is the development of esophagitis, which is inflammation of the esophagus. This can occur when stomach acid irritates the lining of the esophagus, leading to a range of symptoms, including pain, difficulty swallowing, and heartburn.

Over time, untreated acid reflux can lead to a condition called Barrett's esophagus, which occurs when the cells in the lining of the esophagus begin to change. While the condition is not serious in and of itself, it can lead to an increased risk of developing esophageal cancer.

In rare cases, acid reflux can also cause respiratory problems, such as chronic coughing, wheezing, or even pneumonia. This occurs when stomach acid refluxes into the lungs, causing irritation and inflammation.

In addition to the physical complications associated with acid reflux, there are also a number of lifestyle factors that can be impacted by the condition. Many people who suffer from acid reflux may experience difficulty sleeping due to symptoms like heartburn, which can lead to feelings of fatigue and general malaise. Others may experience social anxiety or depression due to the disruption to their daily routines that the condition can cause.

Finally, it is worth noting that there are a number of risk factors that can increase the likelihood of developing complications from acid reflux. These include being overweight or obese, smoking, drinking alcohol or caffeine, and consuming large meals or eating late at night. Those who have a history of gastrointestinal problems or who take certain medications, such as non-steroidal anti-inflammatory drugs (NSAIDs), may also be at an increased risk for complications associated with acid reflux.

In general, while acid reflux is typically not a serious condition, it is important to seek treatment if you experience persistent symptoms. By working with your healthcare provider, you can better manage your symptoms and minimize the risks and complications associated with acid reflux.

Chapter Twenty-Two

Living with Acid Reflux

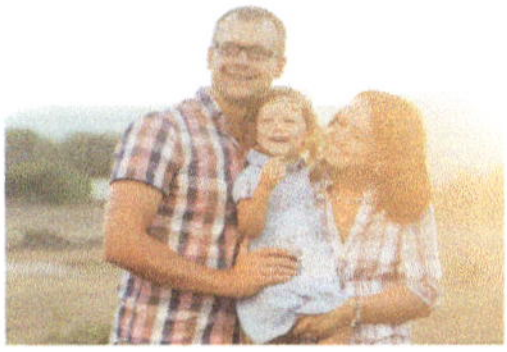

Acid reflux, also known as gastroesophageal reflux disease (GERD), is a chronic condition that can cause discomfort and pain for those who suffer from it. It occurs when stomach acid flows back into the esophagus, causing irritation and inflammation. Living with acid reflux can be challenging, but there are several strategies that can help manage symptoms and improve overall quality of life.

One of the most important things to keep in mind when living with acid reflux is to avoid triggers that can exacerbate symptoms. Common triggers include acidic or spicy foods, fatty or fried foods, caffeine, alcohol, and carbonated beverages. It can be helpful to keep a food diary to identify which foods and drinks tend to cause symptoms, and then make adjustments to your diet accordingly.

In addition to dietary changes, there are several lifestyle modifications that can help alleviate symptoms of acid reflux. For example, it is recommended to eat smaller, more frequent meals instead of large meals, which can put pressure on the lower esophageal sphincter (LES) and contribute to acid reflux. It is also important to avoid lying down or going to bed for at least three hours after eating, as this can increase the risk of acid reflux.

Certain sleeping positions can also be helpful in managing acid reflux symptoms. Sleeping with your head elevated can reduce the amount of acid that flows back into the esophagus. This can be accomplished by using a wedge pillow, or by raising the head of the bed by a few inches.

Another important aspect of managing acid reflux is to maintain a healthy weight. Excess weight can put pressure on the stomach and LES, making it more likely that stomach acid will flow back into the esophagus. Regular exercise and a healthy diet can help with weight management, as well as improve overall health.

If lifestyle modifications and dietary changes do not provide sufficient relief, there are several over-the-counter and prescription medications that can help manage acid reflux symptoms. Antacids, H2 blockers, and proton pump inhibitors (PPIs) are all commonly used to treat acid reflux. Your doctor can help determine which medication is right for you, depending on the severity of your symptoms.

In addition to medications, there are several alternative therapies that can be helpful in managing acid reflux symptoms. For example, acupuncture and hypnotherapy have both been shown to reduce symptoms of acid reflux. It is important to talk to your doctor before trying any alternative therapies, to ensure that they are safe and effective for you.

Living with acid reflux can be challenging, but with the right strategies in place, it is possible to manage symptoms and improve overall quality of life. By avoiding triggers, making lifestyle modifications, and working with your doctor to find the right medication and alternative therapies, you can take control of your acid reflux and live a healthier, more comfortable life.

Chapter Twenty-Three

Frequently Asked Questions.

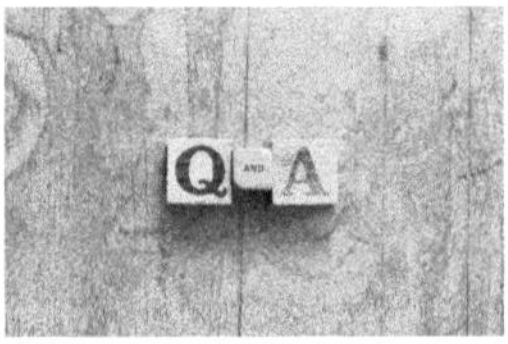

acid reflux

Acid reflux, also known as heartburn or gastroesophageal reflux disease (GERD), is a condition where the contents of the stomach flow back up into the esophagus. This can cause a burning sensation in the chest or throat, as well as nausea, coughing, and other symptoms. There are a number of lifestyle changes you can make to reduce the symptoms of acid reflux, such as avoiding trigger foods, eating smaller meals, and avoiding eating late at night. You can also try over-the-counter medications to reduce stomach acid production or help to keep the contents of your stomach from flowing back up into your esophagus. In some cases, surgery may be necessary to correct the underlying condition.

gastroesophageal reflux

Gastroesophageal reflux (GERD) is a condition in which the acidified liquid content of the stomach backs up into the esophagus. The symptoms of uncomplicated GERD are: heartburn and regurgitation. Heartburn is a burning sensation in the retrosternal chest that occurs when acid refluxes from the stomach into the esophagus. Regurgitation is the sensation of liquid coming up into the back of the throat or mouth.

ger

Acid reflux, also known as GERD, is a condition in which stomach acid flows back up into the esophagus, causing a burning sensation in the chest or throat. GERD is a common condition, affecting up to 20% of the population. There are a variety of treatments available, but some people may require surgery.

heartburn

Heartburn, also known as acid reflux, is a condition in which the acidified liquid content of the stomach backs up into the esophagus. The symptoms of heartburn include chest pain, burning in the throat, and abdominal discomfort. Heartburn can be caused by several factors, including overeating, obesity, pregnancy, smoking, and certain medications. Treatment for heartburn typically involves lifestyle changes, such as avoiding trigger foods and eating smaller meals. In some cases, antacids or other medications may be necessary.

The conclusion of this essay might discuss the fact that acid reflux is a condition that cannot be cured, but can be controlled with medication and lifestyle changes. It might also discuss how this condition can negatively impact a person's life if it is not controlled.

How do I get rid of my acid reflux?

There are a number of things you can do to get rid of your acid reflux. First, you can try over-the-counter antacids or H2 blockers. These medications can help to neutralize the acid in your stomach and help to reduce the symptoms of acid reflux. If you find that these medications do not work well for you, you may want to consider some lifestyle changes. Avoiding Trigger Foods and eating smaller, more frequent meals can help to reduce the symptoms of acid reflux. Finally, if you are still struggling with acid reflux, you may want to talk to your doctor about the possibility of taking a proton pump inhibitor. Proton pump inhibitors can help to block the production of stomach acid, which can provide significant relief from acid reflux.

What triggers acid reflux?

There are a few things that can trigger acid reflux, and they vary from person to person. Some of the more common triggers are eating certain foods, lying down after eating, bending over, and wearing tight clothing. Certain foods are more likely to trigger acid reflux than others. Some of these foods include spicy or fried foods, tomatoes, citrus fruits, chocolate, and garlic. If you find that certain foods trigger your acid reflux, it's best to avoid them. Lying down after eating can trigger acid reflux. This is because gravity helps to keep the stomach acid in the stomach, instead of letting it rise up into the esophagus. Bending over can also trigger acid reflux. This is because the pressure from the stomach can push the acid up into the esophagus. Wearing tight clothing can trigger acid reflux. This is because tight clothing can put pressure on the stomach, which can then push the acid up into the esophagus. There are a few things that can trigger acid reflux. Some of the more common triggers are eating certain foods, lying down after eating, bending over, and wearing tight clothing. If you find that certain foods or activities trigger your acid reflux, it's best to avoid them.

How do you feel when you have acid reflux?

Acid reflux is a condition in which the contents of your stomach come back up into your esophagus, or swallowing tube. This can happen when the muscle that separates your stomach from your esophagus relaxes too much or weakens. Acid reflux can cause a burning sensation in your chest or throat. This is called heartburn. It can be a really unpleasant feeling. You may also have a sour or bitter taste in your mouth. This is caused by the acid from your stomach going up into your throat. Acid reflux can also cause other symptoms. These can include: -A feeling like food is stuck in your throat -Wheezing or coughing -An asthma attack -Changes in your voice -Trouble swallowing If you have acid reflux, you may not necessarily feel all of these symptoms all the time. Some people only get heartburn when they eat certain foods. Others may only get heartburn at night. Acid reflux is usually not a serious condition, but it can be uncomfortable. Some people have it on a daily basis. If you have acid reflux more than twice a week, you may have what is called "gastroesophageal reflux disease" (GERD). This is a more serious condition that can lead to other problems, such as an increased risk of esophageal cancer. If you think you may have acid reflux, talk to your doctor. They can help you figure out what is causing your symptoms and how to treat them.

What are the 4 types of acid reflux?

There are four types of acid reflux: upper abdominal pain, burning sensation in the chest, regurgitation, and difficulty swallowing. Upper abdominal pain is the most common symptom of acid reflux. It is often described as a burning sensation in the chest, and may be accompanied by a sour taste in the mouth. Burning sensation in the chest is another common symptom of acid reflux. This may be felt as a burning sensation behind the breastbone, or as a sharp pain in the center of the chest. Regurgitation is another common symptom of acid reflux. This occurs when stomach acid is regurgitated into the esophagus, causing a sour taste in the mouth. Difficulty swallowing is the most serious symptom of acid reflux. This may be due to a narrowing of the esophagus, or to damage to the esophageal lining. Difficulty swallowing can lead to weight loss and malnutrition.

Does water help with acid reflux?

There is no one-size-fits-all answer to this question, as the best way to manage acid reflux may vary from person to person. However, drinking water is often recommended as a way to help keep symptoms under control. Acid reflux occurs when stomach acid flows back up into the esophagus. This can cause heartburn, chest pain, and other symptoms. Many people find that lifestyle changes, such as avoiding trigger foods and eating smaller meals, can help to reduce symptoms. Drinking plenty of water is also often recommended as a way of managing acid reflux. Water can help to dilute stomach acid, making it less likely to flow back up into the esophagus. It can also help to keep the digestive system hydrated and working properly. aim to drink eight glasses of water per day, or more if you are experiencing symptoms. If you find that your acid reflux is not improving with lifestyle changes and increased water intake, speak to your doctor. There are a range of medications that can be used to treat acid reflux, and your doctor will be able to advise you on the best course of treatment for your individual case.

How quickly does acid reflux go away?

Acid reflux can be a uncomfortable and dangerous condition if left unchecked. So, how quickly does acid reflux go away? Acid reflux occurs when stomach acid flows back up into the esophagus, the tube that connects the throat to the stomach. This can happen when the muscles that ordinarily keep stomach acid in the stomach relax or when the stomach is distended with food. Acid reflux can also happen if the person has a hiatal hernia, which is when part of the stomach protrudes through the opening in the diaphragm that separates the chest and abdominal cavities. Symptoms of acid reflux include heartburn, chest pain, trouble swallowing, a sour taste in the mouth, and regurgitation. If left untreated, acid reflux can damage the esophagus and even lead to cancer. There are a number of things that can be done to treat acid reflux and prevent it from happening in the first place. Avoiding trigger foods, eating small meals, and avoiding lying down immediately after eating can all help. Over-the-counter antacids can also be helpful in relieving symptoms. For people who experience acid reflux regularly, there are a number of prescription medications that can be used to treat the condition. These include proton pump inhibitors and H2 blockers. Surgery is also an option for people who have not found relief with other treatments. If you think you may be experiencing acid reflux, it is important to talk to your doctor so that the cause can be determined and proper treatment can be started.

How do you know if your acid is high?

Acid reflux, also called GERD or heartburn, is experienced when stomach acid flows back up into the esophagus. This can cause a burning sensation in the chest or throat, and people often describe it as "food coming back up." There are a few ways to tell if you have high acid levels in your stomach. First, you may experience frequent heartburn. This is the most common symptom of acid reflux and is usually described as a burning sensation in the chest or throat. Second, you may have acid reflux that causes you to vomit. This can be especially concerning if you vomit blood or food that looks like coffee grounds. Third, you may have difficulty swallowing. This is because the acid can irritate the esophagus and make it difficult to swallow. Fourth, you may experience pain in the abdomen. This is because the stomach acid can cause inflammation in the stomach. Finally, you may have wheezing or coughing. This is because the acid can irritate the lungs and cause wheezing or coughing. If you have any of these symptoms, it's important to see a doctor. They can help you figure out if you have acid reflux and recommend treatment.

Acid reflux occurs when the contents of your stomach come back up into your esophagus. This can happen if the muscle that separates your stomach and esophagus relaxes too much or if your stomach produces too much acid. Acid reflux can cause heartburn, chest pain, and regurgitation. If you have acid reflux, you may need to change your diet, take medication, or have surgery.

Is Milk good for acid reflux?

It is a common myth that milk is good for acid reflux. However, there is no scientific evidence to support this claim. In fact, milk may actually make acid reflux worse. Acid reflux occurs when stomach acid flows back up into the esophagus. This can happen after eating a large meal or drinking a caffeinated beverage. When the stomach acid enters the esophagus, it can cause a burning sensation. Milk may temporarily relieve the symptoms of acid reflux. However, it will not prevent the condition from recurring. Milk may also make the symptoms worse. There are a few reasons why milk may make acid reflux worse. First, milk contains a high amount of fat. Fat slows down the digestion process and can increase the amount of time that stomach acid remains in the esophagus. Second, milk contains calcium. Calcium can bind to stomach acid and make it more difficult to be expelled from the body. This can lead to a build-up of stomach acid and an increased risk of acid reflux. If you are struggling with acid reflux, it is best to avoid milk. There are many other foods and beverages that can provide relief from the symptoms of acid reflux.

Why am I getting acid reflux every day?

Around 60 million adults in the US suffer from acid reflux, also known as GERD. This figure is on the rise, and according to some estimates, as many as 20% of Americans could be affected by 2030. So why is this happening? There are numerous factors that can contribute to acid reflux. One of the most common is diet. Foods that are high in fat, spice, or acid can trigger reflux. Eating large meals, lying down after eating, and eating late at night can also contribute. Other factors include obesity, pregnancy, smoking, and certain medications. Obesity increases the pressure on the stomach, making it more likely for acid to be pushed back up into the esophagus. Pregnancy does the same thing. Smoking relaxes the muscles that keep the stomach closed, and certain medications (such as ibuprofen) can also cause reflux. So what can you do about it? There are a few lifestyle changes you can make to reduce your chances of getting acid reflux. Avoiding trigger foods, eating smaller meals, and avoiding lying down after eating can all help. Losing weight, if you are overweight, can also make a big difference. If you smoke, quitting is the best thing you can do for your overall health, and it will also help with your acid reflux. There are also medications that can help. Antacids can neutralize stomach acid and provide temporary relief. H2 blockers reduce the production of stomach acid, and proton pump inhibitors block the pumps that produce stomach acid. These medications can provide relief, but they don't address the underlying causes of acid reflux. If you're struggling with acid reflux, talk to your doctor. They can help you figure out what's causing your symptoms and develop a treatment plan.

What is the difference between heartburn and reflux?

Heartburn and acid reflux are often used interchangeably, but they are actually two different things. Heartburn is a symptom of acid reflux, which is when stomach acid rises into the esophagus. Reflux can also cause other symptoms, such as regurgitation, difficulty swallowing, and chest pain. Heartburn occurs when the muscle at the top of the stomach, which is called the lower esophageal sphincter, relaxes and allows stomach acid to flow back up into the esophagus. This can happen after eating, or when lying down or bending over. Heartburn is a burning sensation in the chest that can be accompanied by a sour taste in the mouth, difficulty swallowing, or coughing. Acid reflux is a condition in which stomach acid rises into the esophagus. This can happen when the lower esophageal sphincter muscle relaxes or when the stomach is agitated, such as after eating a large meal. Acid reflux can cause heartburn, as well as other symptoms such as regurgitation, difficulty swallowing, and chest pain. Acid reflux is a common condition that affects many people.

How do I test for acid reflux?

There are a few ways to test for acid reflux. The most common test is the pH test. This test measures the level of acidity in your esophagus. A pH level of 7 is neutral, while a level below 7 is acidic. A pH level above 7 is alkaline. If your esophagus is more acidic than neutral, you may have acid reflux. Another way to test for acid reflux is the barium swallow test. This test involves drinking a liquid that contains barium. The barium will help your esophagus show up on an X-ray. If you have acid reflux, the barium will be visible in your esophagus. You may also have a endoscopy to check for acid reflux. During an endoscopy, a doctor will insert a small camera down your throat. The camera will allow the doctor to see your esophagus and stomach. If you have acid reflux, the doctor will be able to see damage to your esophagus. If you think you may have acid reflux, it is important to talk to your doctor.Your doctor will be able to determine if you have acid reflux and develop a treatment plan.

What are the red flags for acid reflux?

There are a few red flags that may indicate that a person has acid reflux. One red flag is if a person experiences heartburn regularly, particularly after eating. Other red flags may include regurgitation, difficulty swallowing, throat pain or discomfort, and cough or wheezing. If a person has any of these symptoms, it is important to see a doctor to get a diagnosis.

How do you know if your acid reflux is serious?

Acid reflux, also known as heartburn, is a burning sensation in the chest that can extend to the neck, jaw, and back. It is often caused by the regurgitation of gastric acid into the esophagus, which can lead to inflammation and irritation of the esophageal lining. While acid reflux is not usually a serious condition, it can be uncomfortable and may cause complications if left untreated. There are a few key symptoms to look out for that may indicate acid reflux. These include heartburn, chest pain, difficulty swallowing, and regurgitation. Acid reflux is often worse at night, and may be accompanied by a sour taste in the mouth or throat. If you experience any of these symptoms regularly, it is important to see your doctor to rule out other potential causes. Acid reflux can often be managed through lifestyle changes, such as avoiding trigger foods, eating smaller meals, and avoiding eating late at night. In some cases, medications may be necessary to control the symptoms. If lifestyle changes and medication do not improve the symptoms, surgery may be recommended. If you think you may be suffering from acid reflux, it is important to see your doctor for a diagnosis. They will likely recommend lifestyle changes and may prescribe medication. If your symptoms are severe or do not improve with treatment, surgery may be an option.

Can acid reflux be something serious?

Acid reflux can be something serious. It is a condition where the acids in your stomach come up into your esophagus. This can cause heartburn and damage to your esophagus. If you have acid reflux, you may need to see a doctor to get it treated.

Acid reflux is a condition in which acid from the stomach flows back up into the esophagus, causing heartburn and other symptoms. It can be treated with lifestyle changes, over-the-counter medications, and prescription medications.

What drinks are good for acid reflux?

There are a few drinks that can help alleviate the symptoms of acid reflux. Milk is a common go-to drink for many people when they're feeling the burn of acid reflux, as it can help coat the stomach and line the esophagus. However, whole milk may actually make your symptoms worse, as the fat content can trigger reflux. Try opting for skim milk instead. Another type of drink that can be helpful is herbal tea. Herbal tea can soothe the digestive system, which can be beneficial if you're dealing with frequent heartburn. Chamomile and ginger tea are particularly good choices. You can also try adding a bit of honey to your tea, as this can help with the soothing process. If you're looking for a non-dairy alternative to milk, you can try almond milk. Almond milk is less likely to cause symptoms of acid reflux than whole milk, as it's lower in fat. It's also a good source of calcium, which can be helpful in keeping your bones strong. If you're trying to avoid caffeine, decaffeinated coffee and herbal tea are both good choices.

However, it's important to note that decaf coffee still contains a small amount of caffeine. If you're sensitive to caffeine, it might be best to avoid it altogether. When it comes to alcohol, moderation is key. Alcohol can relax the esophageal sphincter, which can cause acid reflux. If you do choose to drink, opt for clear liquors like vodka or gin, as they're less likely to trigger symptoms. When it comes to carbonated drinks, it's best to avoid them altogether. The bubbles in carbonated beverages can cause your stomach to bloat, which can put pressure on the sphincter and trigger acid reflux. If you're dealing with frequent heartburn, it's important to talk to your doctor. There are a variety of medications that can be helpful in managing acid reflux. While there are a few drinks that can help with acid reflux, it's important to remember that everyone is different. What works for one person may not work for another. It's important to experiment to see what works best for you.

Is Coke good for acid reflux?

Coke is often thought of as a refreshing drink, but for those who suffer from acid reflux, it can be a nightmare. The carbonation in Coke can cause stomach acid to rise up into the esophagus, leading to pain and discomfort. Coke is not the only beverage that can trigger acid reflux. Other carbonated drinks, such as lemonade and soda, can also cause problems. alcoholic beverages, such as beer and wine, can also contribute to acid reflux. There are a few things that you can do to help lessen the chances of Coke causing you acid reflux. First, try drinking Coke with a straw. This will help to keep the liquid from coming in contact with your teeth, which can cause the stomach acid to rise. Another thing you can do is to drink Coke after a meal, rather than before. This will give your stomach time to digest the food before the Coke hits it and causes the acid to rise. If you find that Coke is still giving you problems, there are some other options you can try. Ginger ale or chamomile tea can sometimes help to soothe the stomach and prevent acid reflux. There are also some medications that can help to control acid reflux. If you find that over-the-counter antacids are not helping, you may want to talk to your doctor about prescription options. Coke can be a trigger for acid reflux, but there are things you can do to help prevent it. If you find that you are still having problems, talk to your doctor about other options that may be available to you.

Is Yogurt good for acid reflux?

Yogurt is often thought of as a healthy food, but for people suffering from acid reflux, it can be a trigger food. Acid reflux is a condition in which stomach acid rises up into the esophagus, causing a burning sensation in the chest or throat. Some people are more sensitive to this than others, and for some, even a small amount of yogurt can cause symptoms. There is no definitive answer as to whether or not yogurt is good for people with acid reflux. Some people find that yogurt soothes their symptoms, while others find that it makes them worse. The best way to determine whether or not yogurt is a trigger food for you is to keep a food diary. Write down everything you eat and drink, as well as when you experience symptoms. If you notice that your symptoms seem to be worse after eating yogurt, it's probably best to avoid it. There are many different types of yogurt, so even if you find that yogurt is a trigger food for you, there may be another type that doesn't cause symptoms. For example, goat's milk yogurt is sometimes easier to digest than cow's milk yogurt. You might also try yogurt that is low in fat or lactose-free. If you enjoy eating yogurt and don't want to give it up entirely, there are a few things you can do to minimize the risk of symptoms. Try eating yogurt with live and active cultures, as these may help to reduce the amount of acid in your stomach. You should also avoid eating yogurt right before bed, as lying down can make symptoms worse. Finally, be sure to choose yogurt that is not too tart or acidic.

When should I go to the doctor for acid reflux?

Acid reflux, also calledGERD, is a common condition where stomach acid rises up into the esophagus. This can cause a burning sensation in the chest or throat, and can sometimes be accompanied by a sour taste in the mouth. Acid reflux is generally considered to be a nuisance, but it can occasionally lead to more serious problems such as Barrett's esophagus or even esophageal cancer. Most people with acid reflux can manage their condition with lifestyle changes and over-the-counter medications. However, there are some cases where acid reflux is severe and does not respond to these treatments. If you are experiencing severe acid reflux, it is important to see a doctor to rule out any other potential problems and to get started on a treatment plan. There are a few different medical tests that can be used to diagnose acid reflux, but the most common is an endoscopy. This procedure involves inserting a small camera down the throat so that the doctor can get a close look at the esophagus. An endoscopy can usually be done on an outpatient basis and does not require any special preparation. If you are experiencing any symptoms of acid reflux, it is important to talk to your doctor. He or she can help you determine if your symptoms are indeed caused by acid reflux and can develop a treatment plan that is right for you.

Can acid reflux heal itself?

The short answer to this question is 'no'. However, there are treatments available that can significantly reduce the symptoms of acid reflux and, in some cases, may even cure the condition. Acid reflux is caused when stomach acid rises up into the esophagus. This can happen for a number of reasons, including a weakened lower esophageal sphincter (LES), pregnancy, excess weight, smoking and certain medications. While there are lifestyle changes that can help reduce the occurrences of acid reflux episodes, unfortunately the condition cannot heal itself. There are a number of different medications that can be used to treat acid reflux. Antacids work by neutralizing stomach acid and can provide relief from occasional heartburn. H2 blockers reduce the amount of acid produced by the stomach and can be taken before meals to prevent heartburn. Proton pump inhibitors (PPIs) are the most effective type of medication for acid reflux as they work to block acid production altogether. Making lifestyle changes such as eating smaller meals, avoiding trigger foods, remaining upright for a few hours after eating and not smoking can also help to reduce the symptoms of acid reflux. In some cases, these changes may be enough to control the condition. For others, medication may still be necessary even with lifestyle changes in place. If you are struggling with acid reflux, it's important to talk to your doctor about your symptoms and treatment options. With proper treatment, you can control the symptoms and enjoy your life.

Does burping make acid reflux worse?

There is no simple answer to whether or not burping make acid reflux worse. It seems that for some people, burping can make their acid reflux worse, while for others, it can actually help to relieve their symptoms. Acid reflux is caused when stomach acid flows back up into the esophagus. This can happen when the lower esophageal sphincter (LES) muscle relaxes or weakens, or when there is pressure on the stomach. Burping can sometimes make acid reflux worse because it can cause the stomach acid to flow back up into the esophagus. If you have acid reflux, you may want to avoid or limit your intake of highly carbonated beverages, as they can also lead to more burping. There are a few other things that you can do to help reduce the symptoms of acid reflux, such as avoiding trigger foods, eating smaller meals, and avoiding lying down for at least three hours after eating. If your symptoms are severe, you may want to talk to your doctor about taking medication to help relieve your symptoms.

How can I test my stomach acid at home?

There are a few simple tests you can do at home to test your stomach acid levels. One of the most common is the 'lemon test'. To do this, simply mix together 1/4 cup of water with 1/4 cup of freshly squeezed lemon juice. Drink this on an empty stomach first thing in the morning and then wait 30 minutes before eating or drinking anything else. If you find that you feel better after drinking this mixture, it is likely that your stomach acid levels are low and you may benefit from taking a supplement. Another simple test you can do at home is the 'vinegar test'. To do this, mix 1 tablespoon of apple cider vinegar with 1 cup of water and drink it on an empty stomach. Again, wait 30 minutes before eating or drinking anything else. If you find that you feel better after drinking the vinegar mixture, it is likely that your stomach acid levels are low and you may benefit from taking a supplement. If you are unsure about your stomach acid levels, or if you are experiencing any other digestive problems, it is always best to speak to a doctor or a registered dietitian.

In conclusion, acid reflux is a condition that affects many people. While there are many over-the-counter and prescription medications available to treat the symptoms of acid reflux, there are also many home remedies that can be effective in reducing the symptoms. If you are suffering from acid reflux, it is important to talk to your doctor to find the best treatment plan for you.

Does stress cause acid reflux?

There's no single answer to this question. While stress may not be a direct cause of acid reflux, it can contribute to it. When you're stressed, your body produces more of the stress hormone cortisol. This hormone is known to promote the production of stomach acid. So, while stress may not be the root cause of your acid reflux, it can make it worse. Acid reflux is a common condition that affects millions of people worldwide. It's characterized by a burning sensation in the chest or throat, and sometimes it can be accompanied by a sour taste in the mouth. Acid reflux is caused when stomach acid flows back up into the esophagus. There are a number of things that can contribute to acid reflux, including a diet high in acidic foods, obesity, smoking, and stress. While there is no one-size-fits-all solution to acid reflux, there are some lifestyle changes you can make to help reduce the symptoms. If you're experiencing acid reflux, it's important to talk to your doctor. They can help you identify the underlying cause and recommend the best course of treatment. In some cases, acid reflux can be a sign of a more serious condition, such as gastroesophageal reflux disease (GERD) or a hiatal hernia.

Are bananas good for acid reflux?

The question of whether bananas are good for people with acid reflux is a controversial one. Some people say that bananas can help ease the symptoms of acid reflux, while other people believe that they can make the condition worse. There is no definitive answer to the question of whether bananas are good for acid reflux. However, there is some evidence to suggest that they may help to relieve the symptoms of the condition. One study found that people with acid reflux who ate a banana every day for one month had a significant reduction in the frequency of their symptoms. Another study found that people with acid reflux who ate a banana every day for two weeks had a significant reduction in the severity of their symptoms. There is also anecdotal evidence to suggest that bananas can help to ease the symptoms of acid reflux. Many people who suffer from the condition say that eating a banana can help to reduce the pain and discomfort that they feel. So, while there is no definitive answer to the question of whether bananas are good for acid reflux, there is some evidence to suggest that they may help to relieve the symptoms of the condition.

What foods to avoid if you have acid reflux?

Acid reflux is a condition in which the stomach contents flow back up into the esophagus, causing heartburn and other symptoms. Avoiding certain foods can help prevent or relieve symptoms. Some foods that may trigger acid reflux include: fatty or fried foods, chocolate, coffee, tea, soda, spicy foods, citrus fruits, tomatoes, onions, and garlic. eating large meals, lying down after eating, and eating within two hours of going to bed can also trigger symptoms. Certain foods can help neutralize stomach acids and help prevent symptoms. These include: bananas, rice, oatmeal, applesauce, and toast. Some people find that drinking milk or taking antacids can also help. If you suffer from acid reflux, it is important to make changes to your diet. Avoiding trigger foods can help control your symptoms. Eating foods that help neutralize stomach acids can also be helpful. If you find that your symptoms are severe or are not relieved by dietary changes, you should speak to your doctor.

Is Bread good for acid reflux?

There are a lot of different opinions out there about whether bread is good or bad for people with acid reflux. Some people say that bread is fine, as long as it's not too greasy or spicy. Others say that bread is a no-no, and that greasy foods are the real culprits. So, what's the truth? Well, it turns out that there isn't a straightforward answer. It really depends on the individual. Some people find that bread doesn't trigger their acid reflux, while others find that it does. There are a few things to keep in mind if you're trying to figure out whether bread is a friend or foe when it comes to acid reflux. First, it's important to remember that everyone is different, and what works for one person may not work for another. Second, it's worth considering the type of bread you're eating. If you're eating a sourdough bread, for example, it's likely to be more tolerable than a white bread, which is more likely to be acidic. In general, it's a good idea to experiment and see how your body reacts to different types of bread. You may find that you can eat a piece of sourdough bread without any problems, but that a white bread sets off your acid reflux. Or, you may find that bread is fine in moderation, but that eating too much of it can trigger your symptoms. If you're struggling with acid reflux, it's important to talk to your doctor. They can help you figure out what's triggering your symptoms and develop a treatment plan that will work for you.

Does empty stomach cause acid reflux?

There are many things that can cause acid reflux, but one potential cause is an empty stomach. When you have acid reflux, it means that your stomach acid is coming up into your esophagus. This can happen when your stomach is empty, because there is nothing there to absorb the acid. There are a few ways to prevent acid reflux, and one of them is to make sure that you eat regularly. Eating small meals throughout the day can help to keep your stomach from getting too empty, and it can also help to keep the acid production under control. There are also certain foods that can help to reduce acid reflux, and you should avoid foods that trigger your symptoms. If you think that empty stomach might be causing your acid reflux, you can try eating a small snack before bedtime. This can help to raise the level of acid in your stomach and reduce the amount of acid that comes up into your esophagus. You should also avoid eating late at night, because this can make your symptoms worse. If you are suffering from acid reflux, you should talk to your doctor. They can help you determine what is causing your symptoms and recommend the best course of treatment.

Can acid reflux make you feel sick?

When you have acid reflux, stomach acid flows back up into your esophagus — the tube that connects your throat to your stomach. This causes a burning sensation in your chest (heartburn). You may also experience a sour or bitter taste in the back of your throat. This is called regurgitation. Acid reflux can cause a variety of symptoms, including: -Heartburn -Regurgitation - Difficulty swallowing - Chest pain - A sour or bitter taste in your throat - Hoarseness - Wheezing - Coughing These symptoms can be aggravated by lying down or bending over. Acid reflux can make you feel sick. Nausea is a common symptom of acid reflux. You may also experience vomiting. This is because the stomach acid irritates your throat and esophagus. If you have acid reflux, you may need to take medication to prevent or relieve your symptoms. Many people with acid reflux can control their symptoms with lifestyle changes, such as avoiding trigger foods and eating smaller meals.

What are the 6 symptoms of heartburn?

Heartburn is a burning sensation in your chest, just behind your breastbone. The feeling can start in your upper abdomen and radiate up into your neck or throat. Heartburn is usually caused by gastroesophageal reflux disease (GERD). GERD is a condition where stomach acid leaks back up into the esophagus. The esophagus is the tube that carries food from your mouth to your stomach. 1. Burning sensation in your chest The most common symptom of heartburn is a burning sensation in your chest. The sensation usually starts behind your breastbone and radiates up to your neck and throat. 2. Discomfort in your upper abdomen Heartburn can also cause discomfort in your upper abdomen. The discomfort may feel like a growling or rumbling noise. It can also cause bloating and make you feel like you have a full stomach. 3. Hiccups Hiccups are a common symptom of heartburn. Hiccups happen when the sphincter muscle at the top of your stomach relaxes, allowing stomach acid to leak back up into your esophagus. 4. Sour taste in your mouth If you have heartburn, you may also taste sour liquid at the back of your mouth. This is called regurgitation. Regurgitation happens when stomach acid leaks back up into your esophagus and esophageal sphincter (the muscle that closes off your throat). 5. Difficulty swallowing Heartburn can make it difficult to swallow. This is called dysphagia. Dysphagia happens when the esophageal muscles are weakened. 6. Pain when you lie down Heartburn is often worse at night. This is because lying down makes it easier for stomach acid to leak back up into your esophagus.

Acid reflux is a serious condition that can cause a lot of pain and discomfort. If you think you may have acid reflux, it is important to see a doctor so they can diagnose and treat the problem. There are many treatments available for acid reflux, so there is no need to suffer.

How do I know if I have indigestion or acid reflux?

Indigestion, also called dyspepsia, is a general term for pain or uncomfortable feelings in the stomach area. Acid reflux is a more serious condition that can cause the contents of the stomach to leak back up the esophagus. Both conditions can cause symptoms such as heartburn, chest pain, and difficulty swallowing. So how can you tell the difference between indigestion and acid reflux? One key difference is that indigestion is often relieved by eating or taking antacids, while acid reflux is not. Acid reflux can also cause symptoms such as nausea, coughing, and a sour taste in the mouth.

If you think you may have acid reflux, it's important to see your doctor to rule out any other potential health problems.

Which tablet is good for acidity?

There are many different types of tablets that can be effective for treating acidity. Some of the most common include antacids, H2 blockers, and proton pump inhibitors. Antacids work by neutralizing stomach acid, while H2 blockers prevent the production of stomach acid. Proton pump inhibitors are the most powerful type of acid-reducing medication, but they can also have the most side effects. Talk to your doctor to determine which type of tablet is right for you.

What causes gastroesophageal reflux disease?

Gastroesophageal reflux disease (GERD) is a condition where stomach contents and acid flow back up into the esophagus. This reflux can cause symptoms such as heartburn and chest pain. GERD is a common condition, affecting about 20% of the US population. There are many possible causes of GERD. One common cause is a malfunctioning lower esophageal sphincter (LES). The LES is a ring of muscle that separates the esophagus from the stomach. Normally, the LES closes tightly after food passes through, but in people with GERD, the LES either opens too often or does not close properly. Another possible cause of GERD is a hiatal hernia. A hiatal hernia occurs when a part of the stomach bulges through an opening in the diaphragm (the muscle that separates the chest and abdominal cavities). This bulge can allow the LES to open more often, leading to GERD. Other possible causes of GERD include: -Certain foods and beverages. Examples include fatty foods, spicy foods, chocolate, coffee, and alcohol. -Smoking. -Obesity. -Pregnancy. -Diseases and conditions that relax the LES or increase the production of stomach acid. Examples include diabetes, scleroderma, and asthma. Treatment for GERD may include dietary changes, lifestyle changes, and medications. People with GERD should avoid foods and beverages that trigger their symptoms. They should also avoid eating large meals, eating late at night, and lying down immediately after eating. lifestyle changes that may help include quitting smoking, losing weight if needed, and elevating the head of the bed 6 to 8 inches. There are also a variety of medications that can treat GERD. Antacids neutralize stomach acid and provide fast, short-term relief. H2 blockers reduce the production of stomach acid and can provide relief for up to 12 hours. Proton pump inhibitors (PPIs) are the most effective type of medication for GERD. They reduce the production of stomach acid and can provide relief for up to 24 hours.

What are the 8 symptoms of GERD?

There are 8 symptoms of GERD, which are: 1. Heartburn 2. Regurgitation 3. Dyspepsia 4. Bloating 5. Belching 6. Water brash 7. Halitosis 8. Chest pain Heartburn is the most common symptom of GERD. It is a burning sensation in the chest that can be severe. It is often worse when lying down or bending over. Regurgitation is another common symptom. This is when acid and food come back up into the throat and mouth. It can be very uncomfortable and may happen after meals. Dyspepsia is a general term for pain or discomfort in the upper abdomen. It is often felt after eating. Bloating is a feeling of fullness in the stomach. This can be caused by gas or eating too much. Belching is the release of gas from the stomach through the mouth. It is often caused by swallowing air. Water brash is a sudden feeling of excess saliva in the mouth. It can be caused by GERD or other conditions. Halitosis is bad breath. It can be caused by GERD or other conditions. Chest pain is a common symptom of GERD. It can be a sharp, burning pain or a dull ache. It is often worse when lying down or bending over.

What are the warning signs of GERD?

Acid reflux, also known as GERD, is a condition where stomach acid flows back up into the esophagus, causing a burning sensation in the chest or throat. This can be a result of a number of different things, such as eating certain foods, lying down after eating, or having a hiatal hernia. GERD can be a mild, occasional problem, or a chronic, life-long condition. There are a few different warning signs that you may have GERD. One of the most common is heartburn. This is a burning sensation in the chest that is often worse after eating or lying down. Other symptoms include regurgitation, trouble swallowing, cough, wheezing, and chest pain. If you experience any of these symptoms, it's important to see your doctor to rule out other potential causes. GERD can often be treated with lifestyle changes, such as avoiding trigger foods, eating smaller meals, and avoiding lying down for at least three hours after eating. In some cases, medication may be necessary to control the symptoms. If you think you may have GERD, talk to your doctor about the best way to manage it.

How serious is gastroesophageal reflux disease?

Gastroesophageal reflux disease (GERD) is a condition in which acid from the stomach flows back up into the esophagus (the food pipe), a situation called reflux. Reflux occurs if the muscles that keep food in the stomach weaken or relax. When this happens, stomach acid can flow back up into the esophagus and cause burning. GERD can be a problem if it's not treated because, over time, the reflux of stomach acid damages the tissue lining the esophagus, causing inflammation and pain. In some cases, it can even lead to precancerous changes in the esophagus. GERD is a common condition, affecting about 20% of the population in the United States. It's most common in adults, but children and infants can also be affected.

GERD is more likely to occur if you're overweight, pregnant, or have a hiatal hernia. There are a number of treatments available for GERD, depending on the severity of the condition. Many people with mild GERD can control their symptoms by making lifestyle changes, such as avoiding trigger foods, eating smaller meals, and not eating close to bedtime. If lifestyle changes don't improve your symptoms, your doctor may recommend medications to reduce the production of acid in your stomach or prevent acid reflux. In some cases, surgery may be necessary to repair the damage to the esophagus. GERD is a serious condition that can have a big impact on your quality of life. If you think you may have GERD, talk to your doctor.

How do you get GERD to go away?

There are a few things you can do to get GERD to go away. For one, you can try over-the-counter medications. These can be very effective in relieving the symptoms of GERD. If these don't work, you can talk to your doctor about prescription medications. There are also some lifestyle changes you can make that can help. quitting smoking, for instance, can be very helpful in reducing the symptoms of GERD. Losing weight if you're overweight can also be helpful. And finally, avoiding certain foods that trigger GERD can also be helpful. These trigger foods vary from person to person, but some common ones include caffeine, chocolate, fatty foods, and spicy foods.

Acid reflux can be a painful and irritating condition, but there are things you can do to help lessen the symptoms. Be sure to consult with your doctor to rule out any other underlying conditions. Avoid trigger foods, eat smaller meals, and elevate your head and chest when sleeping. With a little trial and error, you can find what works best for you to manage your acid reflux.

What is the fastest way to cure GERD?

There are many fast-acting heartburn medications that can relieve GERD symptoms. Antacids work by neutralizing stomach acids. H2 blockers lower acid production. Proton pump inhibitors stop the production of stomach acid. All of these medications can be taken in pill form. There are also liquid and chewable versions of these medications.

Where do you hurt when you have GERD?

When you have GERD, you may experience heartburn, indigestion, chest pain, trouble swallowing, a dry cough, hoarseness, or asthma. Although it may be uncomfortable, GERD is usually not a serious condition. In some cases, however, GERD can lead to more serious problems, such as ulcers, bleeding, or esophageal cancer. GERD occurs when the valve between the stomach and the esophagus, known as the lower esophageal sphincter (LES), does not close properly. This allows stomach acid and food to back up into the esophagus, causing heartburn and other symptoms. There are a number of things that can contribute to the development of GERD, including obesity, pregnancy, smoking, and drinking alcohol. Additionally, certain foods and beverages, such as spicy or acidic foods, citrus fruits, chocolate, caffeine, and mint, can trigger heartburn. If you have GERD, there are a number of things you can do to ease your symptoms. Avoiding trigger foods and beverages, eating smaller meals, and avoiding lying down for three hours after eating can help. Additionally, over-the-counter antacids and medications, such as proton pump inhibitors (PPIs) and histamine-2 (H2) blockers, can be effective in treating heartburn. If you have GERD and your symptoms are not improving with lifestyle changes and over-the-counter medications, you may need to see a doctor. GERD can often be managed successfully with prescription PPIs. In some cases, surgery may be necessary to correct the problem.

Does stress cause GERD?

There are many possible causes of GERD, and one of them is stress. While stress does not directly cause GERD, it can contribute to it by causing changes in the body that make GERD more likely to occur. For example, stress can lead to increased production of stomach acid, which can then lead to GERD. Stress can also cause other changes in the body that can make GERD more likely, such as changes in the way the muscles in the esophagus work. While there is no definitive answer as to whether or not stress causes GERD, it is clear that stress can play a role in making GERD more likely to occur. If you are experience stress, it is important to find ways to manage it in order to help reduce your risk of GERD.

When is GERD an emergency?

Acid reflux is a common condition that affects millions of people worldwide. While most cases of acid reflux are not serious, there are some instances when GERD (gastroesophageal reflux disease) can become an emergency. If you experience any of the following symptoms, you should see a doctor immediately: -Difficulty swallowing -Painful swallowing -Weight loss -Vomiting -Black stools -Choking -Wheezing -Hoarseness If you have any of the above symptoms, it is important to see a doctor right away as they could be indicative of a more serious condition, such as esophageal cancer. While most cases of acid reflux can be managed with lifestyle changes and over-the-counter medications, some cases may require surgery. If you are experiencing acid reflux, it is important to talk to your doctor about your symptoms and treatment options.

What can happen if GERD is left untreated?

GERD, or gastroesophageal reflux disease, is a condition in which stomach contents rise up into the esophagus, sometimes causing symptoms like heartburn, coughing, and trouble swallowing. If left untreated, GERD can lead to serious problems such as Barrett's esophagus, esophageal ulcers, and even esophageal cancer. Barrett's esophagus is a condition in which the lining of the esophagus changes, becoming more like the lining of the intestine. This change is thought to be caused by the repeated exposure to stomach acid that occurs in people with GERD. While Barrett's esophagus is not cancer, it is a risk factor for esophageal cancer. Esophageal ulcers are open sores that form on the lining of the esophagus. They are usually caused by stomach acid, and they can be quite painful. Esophageal ulcers can bleed, and if the bleeding is severe, it can be life-threatening. Esophageal cancer is a rare but serious complication of GERD. The cancer starts in the cells lining the esophagus, and it can spread to other parts of the body. Esophageal cancer is aggressive and difficult to treat. While GERD is a common condition, it is not something to be taken lightly. If you think you may have GERD, see your doctor for an evaluation. Treatment can help to prevent the serious complications that can occur if GERD is left untreated.

Can GERD go away on its own?

GERD, or gastroesophageal reflux disease, is a chronic condition in which the stomach contents, including acid, regurgitate or wash back up into the esophagus. This can cause heartburn, chest pain, and damage to the esophageal lining. GERD is a leading cause of esophageal cancer. While GERD can be a painful and unpleasant condition, it is important to remember that for many people, GERD is a manageable condition. There are a number of lifestyle changes that can help to ease the symptoms of

GERD, and there are also a number of medications that can help to control the condition. For some people, however, GERD may be a more severe condition that requires surgery. Surgery for GERD is generally reserved for those who do not respond to other treatments, and who are at risk for serious complications from the condition. So, can GERD go away on its own? The answer is maybe. For some people, making lifestyle changes may be enough to control the symptoms of GERD and make the condition manageable. For others, however, GERD may be a chronic condition that requires medication or surgery to manage.

Can you get rid of gastroesophageal reflux disease?

The answer to this question is both yes and no. There are treatments that can reduce the symptoms of GERD, but there is no cure. Some people may be able to control their symptoms by making lifestyle changes, such as avoiding foods that trigger reflux or eating smaller meals. Others may need medication to control their symptoms. If you have GERD, you may experience heartburn, indigestion, and a sour taste in your mouth. These symptoms can be caused by a variety of things, but they are most often caused by a malfunctioning of the lower esophageal sphincter (LES). The LES is a muscle that separates the stomach from the esophagus. When this muscle relaxes, stomach acid can flow back up into the esophagus, causing the aforementioned symptoms. There are a number of things that can trigger the relaxation of the LES, including certain foods, obesity, pregnancy, and smoking. Medications such as antacids and proton pump inhibitors can help to reduce the symptoms of GERD by keeping stomach acid in the stomach where it belongs. However, these medications only treat the symptoms and do not address the underlying cause of the disease. Some people may be able to control their symptoms by making lifestyle changes, such as avoiding trigger foods, eating smaller meals, and avoiding late-night meals. Others may need to take medication to control their symptoms. For some people, surgery may be an option.

Acid reflux is a condition that affects millions of people. If left untreated, it can lead to serious health problems. There are many natural and medical treatments available. Talk to your doctor to find the best treatment for you.

Can I drink coffee with GERD?

GERD, also known as gastroesophageal reflux disease, is a condition in which the contents of the stomach regurgitate (back up, or reflux) into the esophagus. This can happen after eating, lying down, or bending over. Common symptoms include heartburn, sour taste in the mouth, and difficulty swallowing. Coffee is a common trigger food for people with GERD. Coffee relaxes the lower esophageal sphincter (LES), which is a muscle that keeps the stomach contents from flowing back up into the esophagus. When the LES is relaxed, stomach acid can more easily flow back up into the esophagus, leading to heartburn and other symptoms. There are a few things you can do to help lessen the symptoms of GERD when drinking coffee. First, try drinking coffee that has been decaffeinated. The caffeine in coffee is what relaxes the LES, so decaf coffee may be less likely to trigger symptoms. Second, drink coffee in small amounts throughout the day instead of all at once. This will help prevent the build-up of stomach acid that can occur when drinking a lot of coffee at once. Finally, avoid adding cream or sugar to your coffee, as these can also trigger symptoms. If you find that coffee is a trigger food for your GERD, there are plenty of other options to choose from. You can try herbal tea, green tea, or decaf tea. There are also a variety of coffee alternatives available, such as chicory coffee and dandelion coffee. Whatever you decide, be sure to listen to your body and avoid anything that seems to make your symptoms worse.

Can lack of sleep cause acid reflux?

There are many things that can cause acid reflux, and one of those things is lack of sleep. When you don't get enough sleep, your body is not able to properly digest food, and this can lead to acid reflux. There are a few reasons why lack of sleep can cause acid reflux. First, when you're sleep-deprived, your body produces more of the stress hormone cortisol. This hormone can lead to inflammation in the gastrointestinal tract, which can then lead to acid reflux. Another reason why sleep deprivation can cause acid reflux is that it can make the muscles in the esophagus weaker. These muscles are responsible for keeping the stomach's contents from flowing back up into the esophagus. When these muscles are weak, it's easier for acid to come back up. If you're struggling with acid reflux, one of the best things you can do is to make sure you're getting enough sleep. If you're not able to get enough sleep, there are a few things you can do to help: - Avoid eating late at night. Eating too close to bedtime can make acid reflux worse. - Try to relax before bed. Taking some time to wind down before sleep can help reduce acid reflux. - Sleep on your left side. Sleeping on your left side can help reduce acid reflux. If you're struggling with acid reflux, lack of sleep may be one of the contributing factors. By making sure you're getting enough sleep, you can help reduce the risk of acid reflux.

What to do when GERD attacks?

When GERD, or acid reflux, attacks, there are a few things you can do to make the pain go away. The first thing you want to do is to sit up. This will help keep the acid down in your stomach. If you are lying down, the acid can come up into your throat and mouth. The next thing you can do is to drink a glass of water. This will help neutralize the acid in your stomach. You can also drink milk or chew on a piece of gum. These will also help to neutralize the acid. If you have antacids, you can take them. This will help to neutralize the acid in your stomach. You can also take over-the-counter medications, such as Pepcid or Zantac. These will also help to neutralize the acid. If the pain is severe, you may want to go to the emergency room. They can give you stronger medications to help neutralize the acid.

When should you get checked for acid reflux?

Acid reflux, also known as gastroesophageal reflux disease (GERD), is a condition in which the contents of the stomach reflux back up into the esophagus. This can cause a variety of symptoms, including heartburn, chest pain, and regurgitation. Acid reflux is generally considered to be a chronic condition, and it can occur at any age. However, there are certain risk factors that can make a person more likely to develop GERD. These include obesity, pregnancy, smoking, and certain medications. If you experience any symptoms of acid reflux on a regular basis, it is important to see your doctor. This is especially true if you experience severe symptoms, such as Chest pain that is not relieved by antacids. recurrent vomiting. difficulty swallowing. weight loss. bleeding from the esophagus. If you have any of these symptoms, please see your doctor as soon as possible. There are a variety of treatments available for acid reflux, and the best course of treatment will vary from person to person. In some cases, lifestyle changes, such as losing weight or quitting smoking, can help to reduce the symptoms of GERD. Additionally, there are a variety of medications that can be used to treat acid reflux, and your doctor can help you to determine which one is best for you. In some cases, surgery may be recommended. If you think that you may be suffering from acid reflux, please see your doctor. With proper treatment, the symptoms of GERD can usually be controlled.

Why do I have acid reflux everyday?

It's estimated that 60 million Americans experience acid reflux at least once a month, and 15 million have it daily. Though acid reflux is most commonly associated with meals like spicy foods, citrus fruits, tomatoes, garlic, and chocolate, pretty much anything we eat can cause symptoms. Even lying down or bending over after a meal can trigger heartburn. There are a few different things that can cause acid reflux. One is a hiatal hernia, which is when the stomach acid and contents backup into the esophagus because the muscle separating the two isn't working properly. This can be caused by obesity, pregnancy, and even smoking. Another cause is eating certain foods. Foods with a lot of acid, fat, or spice can trigger heartburn. Eating large meals or lying down right after eating can also cause symptoms. Drinking alcohol, carbonated beverages, and caffeine can also make heartburn worse. Heartburn can also be caused by some medications like aspirin, ibuprofen, and muscle relaxers. Pregnant women are also more likely to experience heartburn because of the increase in hormones and pressure on the stomach. There are a few things you can do to help relieve heartburn. Avoiding trigger foods, eating smaller meals, and not lying down right after eating can help. Wearing loose clothing and elevating your head while you sleep can also help. Over-the-counter antacids can neutralize stomach acid and provide relief. If you're experiencing heartburn more than a couple of times a week, you should see your doctor.

How do I know if my esophagus is damaged?

There are a few ways to determine if the esophagus is damaged. One way is to look for symptoms of acid reflux. These can include heartburn, chest pain, trouble swallowing, or a feeling like food is stuck in the throat. Additionally, a person may suffer from GERD if they regurgitate blood or have black stools. If these symptoms occur frequently or do not respond to medication, it is important to consult a doctor, as esophageal damage may be present. Another way to tell if there is damage to the esophagus is through an endoscopy. This is a procedure in which a small camera is inserted down the throat in order to take a look at the esophagus. The doctor will be able to see any ulcers, inflammation, or other damage that may be present. A biopsy may also be taken during this procedure in order to confirm a diagnosis. If acid reflux is left untreated, it can lead to serious complication such as esophageal stricture or Barrett's esophagus. Esophageal stricture is a narrowing of the esophagus that can make it difficult to swallow. Barrett's esophagus is a condition in which the lining of the esophagus changes, and it is considered a precancerous condition. Therefore, it is important to seek medical attention if acid reflux is a frequent problem.

How is GERD diagnosed?

Your doctor may recommend a combination of lifestyle changes, medications, and surgical treatments to manage GERD. Lifestyle changes may include: -eating smaller, more frequent meals -avoiding fatty or fried foods, chocolate, caffeine, alcohol, and citrus fruits or juices -giving up smoking -wearing loose-fitting clothes -avoiding lying down for three hours after eating -elevating the head of your bed -losing weight if you're overweight Medications may include: -over-the-counter antacids or medications -prescription drugs such as proton pump inhibitors or H2 blockers Surgical treatments may include: -fundoplication, a surgery to treat GERD -endoscopic techniques -procedures to help strengthen the lower esophageal sphincter If you have symptoms of GERD, your doctor will likely start with a physical exam and a review of your symptoms. If GERD is suspected, your doctor may also recommend one or more of the following tests: - Esophageal pH monitoring: A small tube (catheter) is passed through the nose and positioned in the esophagus. -Esophageal manometry: A small tube is inserted through the nose and positioned in the esophagus. -ambulatory acid (pH) probe test: A small tube is inserted through the nose and positioned in the esophagus. -Upper GI endoscopy: A long, flexible tube with a light and camera attached is passed through the mouth and down the throat. -X-ray of the upper GI tract: A diet of barium is given the night before the test. X-rays are then taken as the barium moves through the esophagus and stomach.

Acid reflux is a condition that affects many people. If you suffer from acid reflux, you know how uncomfortable it can be. There are many treatments available that can help you manage your condition. With the right treatment, you can live a normal, healthy life.

What are the 4 types of GERD?

There are four types of GERD, each with different symptoms. The first type is GERD with esophageal spasm. This type of GERD is characterized by muscle contractions in the esophagus that make it difficult to swallow. The second type is GERD with Barrett's esophagus. This type of GERD is characterized by a change in the tissue lining the esophagus that makes it more susceptible to damage from stomach acid. The third type is GERD with stricture. This type of GERD is characterized by a narrowing of the esophagus that makes it difficult to swallow. The fourth type is GERD with ulcers. This type of GERD is characterized by open sores in the esophagus that are painful and may bleed.

What helps acid reflux at night?

There are a few things you can do to help lessen the symptoms of acid reflux at night. For one, avoid eating large meals or eating late at night. This can help keep the stomach from becoming too full and putting pressure on the lower esophageal sphincter (LES). Another helpful tip is to avoid lying down immediately after eating. Give yourself at least a couple hours to digest before hitting the hay. You can also prop yourself up with pillows while you sleep so that your head and torso are elevated. This can help keep stomach contents from flowing back up into the esophagus. Finally, try wearing loose-fitting clothing and avoid tight belts or waistbands. These can put pressure on your stomach and make reflux more likely. If you follow these simple tips, you may find that your acid reflux symptoms become less bothersome at night. If you have severe symptoms or they don't improve with lifestyle changes, be sure to talk to your doctor. There are also medications that can help reduce acid production or prevent reflux altogether.

Does drinking water help heartburn?

There is anecdotal evidence that drinking water may help to ease the symptoms of heartburn. Heartburn is a common condition that is caused by stomach acid rising up into the esophagus. This can cause a burning sensation in the chest and throat. Drinking water may help to dilute the stomach acid and prevent it from rising into the esophagus. There are a few theories as to why water may help to ease the symptoms of heartburn. One theory is that water can help to neutralize stomach acid. Another theory is that drinking water can help to increase the speed at which stomach acid is emptied into the small intestine. There is no concrete evidence that drinking water is an effective treatment for heartburn. However, it is a safe and inexpensive remedy that may help to ease the symptoms of heartburn for some people. It is important to drink water slowly and avoid drinking large amounts of water all at once. Sipping water throughout the day may be more effective than drinking large quantities of water at once. If you are experiencing frequent or severe heartburn, you should consult with a doctor. Heartburn can be a symptom of a more serious condition, such as gastroesophageal reflux disease (GERD).

What fruit is good for acid reflux?

There are a few different types of fruit that can be helpful for acid reflux. One is bananas. Bananas are a natural antacid, and they can help to relieve some of the symptoms of acid reflux. Another is papaya. Papaya contains enzymes that can help to break down food, and it can also help to reduce acidity in the stomach. Lastly, apples can also be helpful. Apples are high in fiber, which can help to absorb stomach acid and reduce the symptoms of acid reflux.

Acid reflux is a real problem that many people suffer from daily. While antacids can help to neutralize stomach acid, they don't always relieve symptoms. Talk to your doctor if you suffer from frequent acid reflux. They may be able to prescribe a stronger medication. Meanwhile, there are a few things you can do to help lessen symptoms. Avoid triggering foods such as fatty or fried foods. Cut back on caffeine and alcohol. And don't lie down immediately after eating. By making a few simple changes, you can help keep acid reflux under control.

Is GER the same as acid reflux?

Is GER the same as acid reflux? There is a lot of confusion about the terms GER and acid reflux. Some people think that they are the same thing, but they are actually two different conditions. GER (gastroesophageal reflux) is a medical term that is used to describe the movement of stomach contents into the esophagus. This can happen after eating, or when you lie down or bend over. Acid reflux is a more serious condition that is caused by the same thing, but the stomach contents are acid. Acid reflux can cause symptoms such as heartburn, trouble swallowing, and a feeling of food stuck in your throat. GER usually doesn't cause these symptoms. GER is a common condition, and is usually not a cause for concern. However, acid reflux can be a more serious condition. If you have any of the symptoms of acid reflux, you should see a doctor to find out if you have GERD (gastroesophageal reflux disease).

Can GER go away?

GER, or gastroesophageal reflux, is a medical condition that affects the lower esophageal sphincter (LES). The LES is a muscle at the end of the esophagus that opens and closes to allow food and liquid into the stomach. When this muscle relaxes, stomach contents can flow back up into the esophagus. This can cause heartburn and other symptoms. GER is a common condition, and it is often temporary, especially in infants and young children. Most people with GER will not need treatment. Some people may need medication or other treatments to relieve symptoms. In rare cases, GER can lead to more serious problems such as esophagitis (inflammation of the esophagus) or Barrett's esophagus (a precancerous condition). There are several things you can do to reduce the symptoms of GER: • eat smaller meals more often • avoid trigger foods and beverages (such as caffeine, alcohol, and fatty or spicy foods) • avoid eating late at night • prop up your head and shoulders when you sleep • avoid tight-fitting clothing If these lifestyle changes do not help, your doctor may prescribe medication. Medications that can be used to treat GER include antacids, H2 blockers, and proton pump inhibitors (PPIs). These medications can help reduce symptoms by decreasing the amount of acid in the stomach. Surgery is rarely needed to treat GER. GER often improves on its own, especially in infants and young children. If GER does not go away, or if it is causing problems such as heartburn and difficulty swallowing, you should see your doctor.

How do u get rid of heartburn?

There are many ways to get rid of heartburn, and which one is best for you may depend on the severity of your heartburn and other factors. Some simple lifestyle changes can help relieve heartburn, such as avoiding trigger foods, eating smaller meals, and avoiding eating late at night. Some people find relief by elevating the head of their bed. Over-the-counter antacids, such as Tums or Maalox, can help neutralize stomach acid and provide short-term relief. H-2 receptor blockers, such as cimetidine (Tagamet) and ranitidine (Zantac), can decrease the amount of acid your stomach produces and also provide relief. If lifestyle changes and over-the-counter medications don't help, your doctor may prescribe a stronger medication.

When should I be worried about heartburn?

Heartburn is a common problem that can cause a burning feeling in your chest or throat. It is caused by acid reflux, which happens when stomach acid backs up into your esophagus. heartburn is usually worse after you eat or when you lie down. There are some things you can do to ease heartburn, like avoiding trigger foods, eating smaller meals, and avoiding eating late at night. You can also prop yourself up with pillows when you sleep, and avoid wearing tight clothing. If heartburn is persistent and doesn’t go away with home remedies, it could be a sign of a more serious condition called gastroesophageal reflux disease (GERD). GERD is a chronic form of acid reflux that can cause symptoms like heartburn, chest pain, trouble swallowing, and a feeling of a lump in your throat. If you think you might have GERD, it’s important to see your doctor so you can get treatment. Left untreated, GERD can lead to complications like esophageal ulcers and Barrett’s esophagus, which is a precancerous condition. Heartburn is usually nothing to worry about, but if it’s accompanied by other symptoms like chest pain, shortness of breath, or pain in your arm or jaw, it could be a sign of a heart attack. If you experience any of these symptoms, call 911 right away.

What are three symptoms of heartburn?

There are three main symptoms of heartburn: pain in the chest, an acid taste in the mouth, and difficulty swallowing. The pain of heartburn is often described as a burning sensation, and it can vary in intensity from mild to severe. The pain may be worse when you eat, lie down, or bend over. In some cases, heartburn pain can last for several hours. The acid taste in the mouth is often described as sour or acidic, and it can also be accompanied by a burning sensation. Difficulty swallowing can occur when the muscles of the esophagus are not working properly. This can cause food and liquids to back up into the throat and mouth. Difficulty swallowing can also cause pain in the chest and throat.

What drink helps heartburn fast?

There are a few drinks that can help relieve heartburn fast. One is ginger ale, which can help because the ginger can settle the stomach. Another is chamomile tea, which can also help to soothe the stomach. Peppermint tea is another good choice, as the mint can help to relax the muscles in the stomach. Finally, aloe vera juice can also help to calm the stomach and relax the muscles. All of these drinks can help to ease heartburn fast.

Will heartburn go away on its own?

Acid reflux, also known as heartburn, is a condition in which stomach acid rises up into the esophagus. This can cause pain and irritation in the esophagus. Some people may only experience occasional episodes of acid reflux, while others may have it more often. There are a few lifestyle changes that can help reduce the occurrences of acid reflux, such as avoiding spicy or fatty foods, eating smaller meals, and avoiding lying down for three hours after eating. Some people may also need to take medications to help control their acid reflux. In most cases, acid reflux will go away on its own. However, if it becomes a chronic problem, it could lead to more serious health complications. If you are experiencing frequent or severe episodes of acid reflux, you should see a doctor to find out if there is a more serious underlying problem.

Acid reflux can be a painful and disruptive condition, but there are ways to manage it. With lifestyle changes, home remedies, and medication, you can lessen the symptoms of acid reflux and get on with your life.

Is heartburn a red flag?

Is heartburn a red flag? Heartburn is a common symptom of gastroesophageal reflux disease (GERD), which is a condition where stomach acid backs up into the esophagus. Heartburn can be a sign of a more serious condition, such as GERD, and should be evaluated by a doctor. Heartburn is not a red flag for all conditions, but it is important to be aware of the potential causes of your symptoms and to seek medical attention if you experience frequent or severe heartburn.

Is heartburn a symptom of something serious?

Heartburn is a symptom of something serious? Heartburn is a common problem that most people experience at least once in their lives. For some people, heartburn is a mild inconvenience, but for others, it can be a serious problem that needs to be addressed. Heartburn is usually caused by reflux, which is when stomach acid and other contents of the stomach back up into the esophagus. This can happen when the sphincter, a muscle at the end of the esophagus, relaxes too much or when the stomach is full. Heartburn can also be caused by other conditions, such as pregnancy, obesity, and certain medications. Most people experience heartburn occasionally and it is not usually a sign of a serious problem. However, if heartburn is frequent or severe, it may be a symptom of a more serious condition, such as gastroesophageal reflux disease (GERD). GERD is a chronic condition that occurs when stomach acid and other contents of the stomach back up into the esophagus on a regular basis. This can damage the esophagus and cause a variety of symptoms, such as heartburn, trouble swallowing, and chest pain. If you experience heartburn frequently or it is severe, you should see your doctor. They can help to determine the cause of your heartburn and recommend treatment. Treatment for heartburn may include lifestyle changes, such as eating smaller meals and avoiding foods that trigger heartburn. Medications, such as antacids and acid blockers, can also be effective in treating heartburn. In some cases, surgery may be necessary to treat GERD. Heartburn is a common problem, but it can be a sign of a serious condition. If you experience heartburn frequently or it is severe, see your doctor to find out the cause and get treatment.

Does heartburn mean heart trouble?

Acid reflux, also known as heartburn, is a medical condition in which stomach acid rises up into the throat, causing a burning sensation. Many people worry that this means they are at risk for heart disease, but this is not necessarily the case. There are a number of different factors that can contribute to acid reflux, including certain foods and beverages, pregnancy, obesity, and certain medications. In many cases, it is simply a matter of making some lifestyle changes, such as avoiding trigger foods and eating smaller meals. For some people, however, acid reflux is a more serious condition that requires medical treatment. If you experience heartburn more than once a week, or if it is accompanied by other symptoms such as difficulty swallowing, chest pain, or shortness of breath, you should see a doctor. Acid reflux is not a pleasant condition, but it is usually not serious.

With a little lifestyle modification and, in some cases, medical treatment, you can control your symptoms and enjoy your life.

What triggers heartburn?

Heartburn is a common condition that affects many people. The main symptom of heartburn is a burning sensation in the chest, which can be accompanied by a sour taste in the mouth, throat, or abdomen. Heartburn is usually triggered by eating certain foods, drinking alcohol, or smoking. Certain foods can trigger heartburn by irritating the lining of the esophagus or by increasing the amount of acid in the stomach. Common trigger foods include fatty or fried foods, spicy foods, citrus fruits, tomatoes, chocolate, coffee, and alcohol. Eating large meals or lying down shortly after eating can also trigger heartburn. Heartburn can also be triggered by smoking, which irritates the lining of the esophagus and increases the amount of acid in the stomach.Smoking also decreases the pressure in the lower esophageal sphincter (LES), which is a muscle that helps to keep stomach contents from flowing back into the esophagus. Stress can also trigger heartburn. When you're stressed, your body produces more of the hormone adrenaline. Adrenaline can increase the amount of acid in your stomach and make the LES muscle relax, allowing stomach contents to flow back into the esophagus.

What causes sudden heartburn?

Acid reflux is caused by a variety of factors. The most common is a weakened lower esophageal sphincter (LES). The LES is a ring of muscle that helps keep stomach contents from rising up into the esophagus. If the LES is weakened or relaxes too much, stomach acid can rise up into the esophagus and cause heartburn. Other factors that can contribute to acid reflux include: being overweight or obese, lying down after eating a meal, eating spicy, fatty, or acidic foods, drinking alcohol, smoking, and pregnancy. Some medical conditions can also cause or worsen acid reflux, such as hiatal hernia, GERD, and gastritis. Acid reflux usually only causes a problem if it occurs frequently or if it is severe. Many people have occasional heartburn without any other problems. However, if acid reflux occurs more than twice a week, it is considered to be GERD. GERD can lead to more serious problems, such as inflammation of the esophagus, Barrett's esophagus, and ulcers. Treatment for GERD usually includes lifestyle changes, such as eating smaller meals and avoiding trigger foods. Medications, such as antacids, proton pump inhibitors, and H2 blockers, can also be used to reduce the symptoms of GERD.

What's the difference between heartburn and indigestion?

Heartburn and indigestion are often used interchangeably, but they actually have different meanings. Heartburn is a burning sensation in your chest that is often caused by eating spicy or fatty foods. Indigestion, on the other hand, is a general term that describes discomfort in your upper abdomen. This may be accompanied by bloating, nausea, or heartburn. So, what's the difference between heartburn and indigestion? Heartburn is a symptom of indigestion, but not all cases of indigestion include heartburn. Indigestion is a general term that describes discomfort in your upper abdomen. This may be accompanied by bloating, nausea, or heartburn. Heartburn, on the other hand, is a burning sensation in your chest that is often caused by eating spicy or fatty foods.

Does milk help with heartburn?

Heartburn, also known as acid reflux, is a burning sensation in the chest. It is caused by acid from the stomach rising up into the esophagus. Heartburn can be relieved by taking antacids, drinking milk, or eating small meals. Drinking milk is a common home remedy for heartburn. However, there is no scientific evidence to support this claim. Milk may temporarily soothe the esophagus and stop the burning sensation. However, it will not prevent the acid from coming back up. There are a few reasons why milk may help with heartburn. First, milk contains calcium, which can neutralize stomach acid. Second, milk is a buffer, meaning it can help to dilute the acid in the stomach. It is important to note that while milk may provide some relief, it is not a cure for heartburn. If you experience heartburn regularly, you should see a doctor. Heartburn can be a symptom of a more serious condition, such as gastroesophageal reflux disease (GERD) or a heart condition.

Acid reflux is a medical condition that can be extremely uncomfortable for those who suffer from it. Thankfully, there are a number of treatments available that can provide relief. While there is no cure for acid reflux, with proper treatment, most people are able to manage their symptoms and live relatively normal lives.

What gets rid of heartburn at night?

There are a few things that can help get rid of heartburn at night. One is to sleep on your left side. This takes the pressure off of your stomach and prevents acid from coming up. Another is to prop your head up with pillows so that your head is above your stomach. This also prevents acid from coming up. Lastly, you can try antacids. Antacids work by neutralizing the acid in your stomach.

What foods get rid of heartburn?

There are many foods that can help relieve heartburn. Some of these include: -Herbal teas: Herbal teas can help soothe the digestive tract and calm the stomach. Some great options include ginger tea, chamomile tea, and lavender tea. -Yogurt: Yogurt is a great option for those who suffer from heartburn. It is packed with probiotics which can help to heal the digestive tract. -Oatmeal: Oatmeal is a great source of fiber and can help to absorb stomach acid. -Fennel: Fennel is a plant that has a long history of being used to relieve digestive issues. -Green vegetables: Green vegetables are packed with nutrients and can help to alkalize the body. -Almonds: Almonds are a great source of healthy fats and can help to coat the stomach.

Does Gaviscon help with heartburn?

If you suffer from heartburn, you're not alone. In fact, about 60 million Americans experience heartburn at least once a year. Heartburn is caused by acid reflux, which is when stomach acid backs up into the esophagus. Gaviscon is a medication that is used to treat heartburn by neutralizing stomach acid. It is available over-the-counter and does not require a prescription. Gaviscon comes in a liquid or tablet form and is taken after meals and at bedtime. So, does Gaviscon help with heartburn? The answer is yes. Gaviscon can help to relieve heartburn symptoms by neutralizing stomach acid. It is available over-the-counter and does not require a prescription. Gaviscon comes in a liquid or tablet form and is taken after meals and at bedtime. If you suffer from heartburn, give Gaviscon a try. It just might be the relief you're looking for.

How long is too long for heartburn to last?

Heartburn is a symptom of acid reflux, and typically feels like a burning sensation in the chest, often after eating. So, how long is too long for heartburn to last? Unfortunately, there is no easy answer to this question.

Heartburn is considered chronic if it occurs more than twice a week, and can last for weeks, months, or even years. If you experience heartburn regularly, you should see your doctor to rule out any underlying medical conditions. There are a few things you can do to help alleviate heartburn. Avoiding trigger foods, eating smaller meals, and avoiding lying down immediately after eating can all help. Over-the-counter antacids can also help to neutralize stomach acid. If heartburn is a frequent and severe problem, your doctor may prescribe medication to reduce stomach acid production. If you experience heartburn, it is best to see your doctor to rule out any underlying medical conditions. There are a few things you can do to help alleviate heartburn. Avoiding trigger foods, eating smaller meals, and avoiding lying down immediately after eating can all help. Over-the-counter antacids can also help to neutralize stomach acid. If heartburn is a frequent and severe problem, your doctor may prescribe medication to reduce stomach acid production.

Where does it hurt when you have heartburn?

When you have heartburn, it can feel like the sharp, hot pain of a sunburn on your chest. The pain can also spread to your neck, jaw, or ear. You might have trouble swallowing or have the feeling of food stuck in your throat. You might get hoarse when you talk, or you might have a dry, hacking cough. If heartburn is untreated, it can also lead to ulcers, bleeding in the esophagus, and an increased risk of cancer.

When should you not ignore heartburn?

If you experience heartburn more than twice a week, you might have gastroesophageal reflux disease (GERD). Heartburn is the most common symptom of GERD, but other symptoms may include regurgitation, difficulty swallowing, and chest pain. GERD is a chronic condition that can be managed with lifestyle changes and medication. If left untreated, however, GERD can lead to serious complications, such as esophageal strictures or ulcers, Barrett's esophagus, and even esophageal cancer. If you think you might have GERD, it's important to see your doctor for a diagnosis and to talk about your treatment options. There are a variety of medications available to treat GERD, and your doctor can help you choose the one that's right for you. In some cases, lifestyle changes may be enough to manage your symptoms. Avoiding trigger foods, staying upright after eating, and losing weight if you're overweight can all help. Quitting smoking and elevating the head of your bed may also be helpful. If you have heartburn that's not relieved by lifestyle changes or medication, you should see your doctor for further evaluation. Your doctor may recommend additional testing, such as an upper endoscopy, to rule out other possible causes of your symptoms.

Does Covid 19 feel like heartburn?

Covid 19 has a lot of similarities to heartburn. For one, both can cause a burning sensation. Additionally, both can be aggravated by certain foods and beverages. Covid 19 can also cause chest pain, shortness of breath, and coughing, which are all symptoms of heartburn. heartburn is often worse at night, and Covid 19 can also be worse at night. Covid 19 can also cause nausea and vomiting, which are also symptoms of heartburn. So, if you have these symptoms, you may want to see a doctor to rule out Covid 19.

Acid reflux, also called gastroesophageal reflux, can be a painful condition caused by the regurgitation of acidic stomach contents into the esophagus. Often, lifestyle changes, such as avoiding trigger foods and eating smaller meals, can help to manage the symptoms of acid reflux. In some cases, medications may be necessary to control the symptoms. If you are experiencing acid reflux, talk to your doctor to determine the best course of treatment for you.

How do I know if it's just heartburn?

How do I know if it's just heartburn? Heartburn is a common problem that causes a burning sensation in the chest. It is caused by stomach acid flowing back up into the esophagus, the tube that carries food from the mouth to the stomach. Heartburn is also known as acid reflux, and it can be a very uncomfortable experience. The good news is that there are some simple things you can do to ease the discomfort and get rid of the heartburn. If you think you may be experiencing heartburn, the first step is to try to identify the trigger. Common triggers include spicy food, fatty food, citrus, tomatoes, chocolate, caffeine, and alcohol. If you can identify the trigger, it may be possible to avoid it in the future. There are also a number of lifestyle changes you can make that may help to reduce the severity of heartburn. These include losing weight if you are overweight, quitting smoking, and avoiding tight-fitting clothing. If you have heartburn frequently, you may want to talk to your doctor about medications that can help to reduce the acid in your stomach. Over-the-counter antacids are often effective, but if you find yourself using them frequently, you may need a stronger prescription medication. Heartburn is a common problem, but it is important to be aware that it can be a symptom of other, more serious conditions. If you have heartburn and it is accompanied by other symptoms such as shortness of breath, chest pain, or trouble swallowing, you should see a doctor right away.

Can Gaviscon make reflux worse?

There are a lot of different medicines out there that people take for acid reflux, but one of the most popular is Gaviscon. There are a lot of people who swear by it and say that it has helped them immensely. However, there are also a lot of people who say that Gaviscon has made their acid reflux worse. So, can Gaviscon make reflux worse? There is no definitive answer, as it seems to be different for everyone. Some people do find that Gaviscon makes their acid reflux worse, while others find that it doesn't make any difference or even helps to improve their condition. It is thought that Gaviscon may make reflux worse for some people because it can cause constipation. Constipation can cause a build-up of pressure in the abdomen, which can then lead to acid reflux. If you are taking Gaviscon and find that it is making your acid reflux worse, you should speak to your doctor about it. They may be able to prescribe a different medication that will not cause constipation and therefore may be better for you. Acid reflux is a very individual condition and what works for one person may not work for another. If you are struggling to find a medication that works for you, it is important to speak to your doctor so they can help you find the right treatment.

Why wont my heartburn go away?

A burning sensation in your chest (heartburn) that occurs after eating and lasts a couple of hours is the most common symptom of gastroesophageal reflux disease (GERD). Heartburn is caused by stomach acid that backs up into your esophagus (the tube that connects your mouth and stomach). GERD can be uncomfortable. But most people can manage the condition by making lifestyle changes and taking over-the-counter medications. If you have GERD, your first step should be to cut back on your consumption of alcohol, caffeine, chocolate, peppermint, fatty foods, and spicy foods. These can all trigger heartburn. In addition, you should try to avoid eating large meals. Eating smaller meals more often can help reduce the amount of stomach acid that is produced. And don't eat within two hours of lying down; this can allow stomach acid to move back up into your esophagus. You should also try to sleep with your head and chest elevated. This will help to keep stomach acid from moving up into your esophagus while you are asleep. If these lifestyle changes don't help, you may need to take medication. Over-the-counter antacids can help neutralize stomach acid. H2 blockers, such as cimetidine (Tagamet) and ranitidine (Zantac), can decrease the amount of acid your stomach produces. And proton pump inhibitors, such as omeprazole (Prilosec) and lansoprazole (Prevacid), can reduce the amount of acid your stomach produces. If you have GERD, it is important to see your doctor if you are having difficulty managing your symptoms. GERD can lead to serious complications, such as esophageal cancer. But if it is caught early and treated, the risks are much lower.

Can stress cause heartburn?

The experience of heartburn is different for everyone. Some people may feel a burning sensation in their chest or throat, while others may feel like food is coming back up into their mouth. Heartburn is a common symptom of acid reflux, which occurs when stomach acid rises up into the esophagus. There are many different causes of heartburn, but one of the most common is stress. Stress can cause the stomach to produce more acid, and it can also lead to tightness in the chest and throat, which can make heartburn worse. If you're experiencing heartburn, it's important to find ways to manage your stress. There are a few different ways that you can manage stress in your life. Exercise is a great way to relieve stress. Taking a few minutes out of your day to go for a walk, run, or bike ride can help you to clear your head and reduce stress. If you can't get outside, taking a yoga or pilates class can also be helpful. In addition to exercise, another way to reduce stress is to make sure that you're getting enough sleep. When you're tired, your body is under more stress and that can lead to heartburn. Make sure that you're getting at least seven to eight hours of sleep each night. You can also try to reduce stress by taking some time for yourself each day. This can mean taking a few minutes to read your favorite book, taking a baths, or listening to calming music. Whatever you enjoy, taking some time for yourself can help to reduce stress and ease heartburn.

What does severe heartburn feel like?

Acid reflux, or heartburn, is a feeling of burning pain in the chest, just behind the breastbone. The pain is often worse after eating, during pregnancy, or when lying down. Some people have GERD, which is a more serious form of acid reflux. GERD can cause damage to the esophagus over time. Severe heartburn is pain that is so intense that it interferes with your daily activities. The pain may wake you up at night. You may feel like you have food stuck in your throat. GERD can also cause a dry cough, hoarseness, or trouble swallowing. If you have severe heartburn, you should see your doctor. There are treatments that can help.

Does heartburn cause heart attacks?

Acid reflux, also known as heartburn, is a condition in which stomach acid flows back up into the esophagus. This can cause a burning sensation in the chest or throat. Acid reflux is a common condition that affects many people, but it is not clear if it can cause heart attacks. There is no direct evidence that acid reflux causes heart attacks. However, some indirect evidence suggests that there may be a link between the two. One study found that people with acid reflux are more likely to have heart attacks than people without acid reflux. The link between acid reflux and heart attacks is not clear. However, if you have acid reflux, you should see a doctor to rule out other potential causes of heart attacks.

What does trapped gas in chest feel like?

When you have gas trapped in your chest, it can feel like you can't breathe. You may feel like you have to burp or pass gas, but nothing comes out. This can be a very uncomfortable feeling. If you're having trouble breathing, you should see a doctor.

Acid reflux is a common condition that can cause a number of symptoms, including heartburn, indigestion, and chest pain. While there are a number of over-the-counter and prescription medications available to treat acid reflux, there are also a number of lifestyle changes that can be effective in alleviating symptoms. These lifestyle changes include avoiding acidic and spicy foods, quitting smoking, and avoiding eating large meals before bedtime.

Do bananas help heartburn?

Bananas are a great fruit for people suffering from heartburn for a number of reasons. First,Bananas contain natural antacids that can help to soothe the stomach and prevent heartburn. Secondly, Bananas are a great source of dietary fiber, which can help to keep the digestive system working properly and prevent heartburn. Finally, Bananas are also a good source of potassium, which can help to reduce stomach acidity and heartburn.

Is yoghurt good for acid reflux?

There are many different opinions on whether or not yoghurt is good for acid reflux. Some people say that yoghurt can help to reduce the symptoms of acid reflux, while others claim that it can actually make the condition worse. Yoghurt is made from milk that has been fermented by bacteria. The main bacteria used to make yoghurt are Lactobacillus bulgaricus and

Streptococcus thermophilus. These bacteria produce lactic acid, which gives yoghurt its sour taste. Lactic acid is thought to have a number of health benefits, including the promotion of healthy digestion. Some people believe that this means that yoghurt may help to reduce the symptoms of acid reflux. However, it is worth noting that yoghurt also contains a lot of fat. This means that it can actually make the symptoms of acid reflux worse. Fatty foods are one of the main triggers of acid reflux. If you are considering eating yoghurt to help with your acid reflux, it is important to speak to a doctor or dietitian first. They will be able to advise you on whether or not yoghurt is likely to be helpful in your particular case. In general, it is thought that plain, unsweetened yoghurt is the best type to eat if you are trying to avoid triggering acid reflux. However, everyone is different and you may find that you tolerate some types of yoghurt better than others. If you do decide to eat yoghurt to help with your acid reflux, it is important to eat it in moderation. Eating large amounts of yoghurt is likely to make your symptoms worse. It is also important to avoid eating yoghurt late at night, as this is when acid reflux is most likely to happen.

Why am I having so much heartburn at night?

Heartburn is a common problem that can cause a burning feeling in your chest or throat. It can also make you feel like you have a lump in your throat. Heartburn can be a symptom of acid reflux, which is a condition where stomach acid flows back up into your esophagus (the tube that carries food from your mouth to your stomach). There are a few things that can make you more likely to get heartburn at night. For one, lying down makes it easier for stomach acid to flow back up into your esophagus. That's because when you're upright, gravity helps keep stomach acid in your stomach. But when you're lying down, gravity isn't working in your favor. Another reason you might get heartburn at night is because you're eating closer to bedtime. This gives your stomach less time to digest your food before you lie down. And if you're eating a big meal or foods that are high in fat, that can make heartburn more likely. There are a few things you can do to help prevent heartburn at night. One is to eat smaller meals so that your stomach doesn't have to work as hard. And try to avoid foods that are high in fat. You can also try elevating your head with pillows when you sleep. This can help keep stomach acid from flowing back up into your esophagus. If you're still having trouble with heartburn, talk to your doctor. There are medicines that can help. And in some cases, surgery might be an option.

Why is heartburn worse at night?

When you lie down, it's easier for stomach acid to move up into your esophagus — the tube that connects your stomach to your throat. This causes the burning sensation known as heartburn. There are a few reasons why heartburn is worse at night. First, gravity isn't working in your favor. When you're upright, it's easier for your stomach contents to move downward into your intestines. But when you lie down, gravity pulls on your stomach contents in the opposite direction — up into your esophagus. Second, there's less saliva produced at night. Saliva is alkaline, which can neutralize stomach acid. So, less saliva means more stomach acid. Third, your stomach empties more slowly at night. So, there's more time for stomach acid to move up into your esophagus. Fourth, you may be more relaxed at night, which can loosen the muscles that keep stomach acid in its place. There are a few things you can do to ease heartburn at night: * Prop up your head and shoulders with pillows. This will help keep acid in your stomach. * Avoid eating late at night. Give yourself at least three hours to digest before lying down. * Avoid trigger foods. These include fatty foods, spicy foods, citrus fruits, and caffeine. * Eat smaller meals. * Quit smoking. * Wear loose-fitting clothing. Tight clothing can put pressure on your stomach and make heartburn worse.

The causes of acid reflux are many and varied, but most commonly it is caused by a weakened or dysfunctional lower esophageal sphincter (LES), which allows stomach acids to back up into the esophagus. This can be the result of lifestyle choices, such as eating a diet high in fatty or spicy foods, or it can be the result of a medical condition, such as gastroparesis. Acid reflux can also be caused by certain medications, such as aspirin, beta-blockers, and calcium channel blockers. If you suffer from acid reflux, it is important to identify the underlying cause so that you can make the necessary changes to your diet or lifestyle, or start taking the appropriate medication.

How do you fix silent reflux?

There are a few things you can do to fix silent reflux. First, you can try over-the-counter medications. These can help to reduce the amount of stomach acid that is produced. You can also make some lifestyle changes, such as avoiding trigger foods and eating smaller meals more often. Finally, you may need to see a doctor to get a prescription for a stronger medication.

Will silent reflux ever go away?

The question of whether silent reflux will ever go away is a difficult one to answer. There are a number of factors that contribute to the development of silent reflux, and it is not always clear why some people seem to suffer from it more than others. Silent reflux can be a very frustrating condition to live with, but there are a few things that you can do to help manage it. First, it is important to understand what silent reflux is. Silent reflux, also known as laryngopharyngeal reflux (LPR), is a condition in which stomach acid and other digestive fluids flow back up into the throat. This can cause a range of symptoms, including hoarseness, a sore throat, and difficulty swallowing. Silent reflux is different from gastroesophageal reflux disease (GERD) in that it does not always cause heartburn or indigestion. There are a number of lifestyle changes that can help to reduce the symptoms of silent reflux. Avoiding trigger foods, quitting smoking, and managing stress can all help to lessen the frequency and severity of attacks. People with silent reflux may also find relief by sleeping with their head elevated. There are a number of over-the-counter and prescription medications that can also be used to treat silent reflux. Antacids and H2 blockers can help to reduce the amount of acid in the stomach, while proton pump inhibitors can prevent the production of acid altogether. These medications can be very effective, but they should be used under the supervision of a doctor. In some cases, surgical intervention may be necessary to treat silent reflux. This is typically only recommended when other treatment options have failed. Surgery for silent reflux usually involves making a small incision in the throat in order to widen the opening of the esophagus. This can help to prevent stomach acid from flowing back up into the throat. The answer to the question of whether silent reflux will ever go away is not a simple one. For some people, the condition may improve with lifestyle changes and medication. However, others may need to undergo surgery in order to find relief. If you are struggling with silent reflux, it is important to talk to your doctor about the best treatment options for you.

What is the difference between acid reflux and silent reflux?

There are two types of reflux: acid reflux and silent reflux. Acid reflux is when stomach acid flows back up into the esophagus. This can cause heartburn and other symptoms. Silent reflux is when stomach acid flows back up into the throat. This can cause hoarseness, a sore throat, and other symptoms.

What is the main cause of silent reflux?

The main cause of silent reflux is undiagnosed GERD. GERD is a condition where the acid in your stomach backs up into your esophagus. This can happen when you eat certain foods, or when you lie down after eating. The symptoms of silent reflux can be hard to spot, because they often happen at night.

What are the signs of silent reflux?

The signs of silent reflux can be difficult to spot. Many people with silent reflux do not have the traditional symptoms of heartburn or indigestion. Instead, they may have a cough, hoarseness, or trouble swallowing. Other signs include bad breath, a sour taste in the mouth, and a feeling of fullness or bloating. If you think you may have silent reflux, it is important to see a doctor for a diagnosis.

What are the dangers of silent reflux?

The danger of Silent Reflux is that it can lead to serious health problems over time if it is not treated. Left unchecked, Silent Reflux can cause damage to the esophagus and even lead to cancer. Silent Reflux is also linked to other health problems such as sleep apnea and asthma.

Does Gaviscon help with silent reflux?

There is some evidence to suggest that Gaviscon may help with silent reflux. Silent reflux, also known as laryngopharyngeal reflux (LPR), is a type of reflux that occurs when stomach acid and other contents of the stomach flow back up into the larynx (the voice box) and pharynx (the throat). Although silent reflux is similar to gastroesophageal reflux disease (GERD), it often does not cause heartburn or other noticeable symptoms. However, it can cause other symptoms such as hoarseness, vocal cord problems, trouble swallowing, and chronic cough. Gaviscon is a medication that is used to treat heartburn and other types of acid reflux. It works by forming a barrier between the stomach and the esophagus to prevent acid from flowing back up. Gaviscon is available over-the-counter and does not require a prescription. There is some evidence to suggest that Gaviscon may help with silent reflux. A study published in the journal "Laryngoscope" found that Gaviscon was effective in reducing symptoms of silent reflux, including hoarseness, trouble swallowing, and chronic cough. Another study, published in the "European Journal of Gastroenterology and Hepatology," found that Gaviscon was effective in reducing the amount of acid that flowed back up into the esophagus. However, more research is needed to confirm these findings. If you are experiencing symptoms of silent reflux, talk to your doctor. Silent reflux can often be treated with lifestyle changes, such as avoiding triggers, eating smaller meals, and staying upright after eating. Medications, such as Gaviscon, may also be recommended.

Acid reflux, or GERD, is a condition where stomach acid rises up into the esophagus, causing discomfort and damage. While there are many medications available to help control acid reflux, making lifestyle changes is often the best way to prevent and treat the condition. These changes include avoiding trigger foods and drinks, eating smaller meals, and avoiding lying down for 3 hours after eating. Making these simple changes can go a long way in preventing and managing acid reflux.

What is the best medicine for silent reflux?

Acid reflux, also known as gastroesophageal reflux (GERD), is a condition where stomach acid rises up into the esophagus. This can cause heartburn, chest pain, and regurgitation. Silent reflux is a variant of acid reflux that doesn't cause any symptoms. The best medicine for silent reflux is proton-pump inhibitor (PPI). PPIs work by inhibiting the production of stomach acid. This reduces the amount of acid that can rise up into the esophagus, and thus, reduces the risk of heartburn, chest pain, and regurgitation. PPIs are available over-the-counter or by prescription. There are a few things you can do to help reduce the risk of silent reflux. First, avoid trigger foods and drinks. Common trigger foods include fatty foods, spicy foods, citrus fruits, and caffeine. Second, eat smaller meals more frequently throughout the day rather than large meals. Third, elevate your head while you sleep by placing pillows under your head and shoulders. This will help keep stomach acid from rising up into the esophagus. Finally, avoid wearing tight-fitting clothes that can put pressure on your abdomen and cause heartburn. If you think you may have silent reflux, talk to your doctor. They can help you determine the best course of treatment.

How do you test for silent reflux?

Acid reflux is a condition in which stomach acid leaks back up into the esophagus, causing a burning sensation in the chest or throat. Silent reflux, also known as laryngopharyngeal reflux (LPR), is a type of acid reflux that does not cause any symptoms. There are a few ways to test for silent reflux. One method is the barium swallow test, which involves drinking a barium solution and then having an X-ray taken. This test can show whether there is any damage to the esophagus from acid reflux. Another way to test for silent reflux is the pH probe test. This test involves inserting a small tube into the esophagus and then measuring the level of acidity in the esophagus over a period of 24 hours. This test can show whether there is any regular reflux of stomach acid into the esophagus. If you think you may have silent reflux, it is important to talk to your doctor so that the proper diagnosis can be made and appropriate treatment can be started.

What should you avoid with silent reflux?

If you suffer from silent reflux, also known as laryngopharyngeal reflux (LPR), you may not be aware of some of the things that can trigger your symptoms. Many people with LPR are surprised to learn that some of the foods they regularly eat are actually making their reflux worse. In order to get your silent reflux under control, it is important to avoid the following trigger foods: Citrus fruits: Lemons, oranges, and other citrus fruits are loaded with acid, which can contribute to silent reflux. If you love citrus fruits, you may be able to tolerate small amounts if you eat them with other foods that buffer the acidity. Tomatoes: Another acidic fruit, tomatoes are a common trigger food for people with silent reflux. If you can't imagine giving up tomatoes, try eating them in small amounts or cook them to help reduce the acidity. Spicy foods: Spicy foods can be a major trigger for people with silent reflux. If you enjoy spicy foods, try to limit them to occasional indulgences rather than making them a regular part of your diet. Fatty foods: Fatty foods can slow down the movement of food through your digestive system, which can lead to silent reflux. To avoid this, limit your intake of fatty foods or eat them in small amounts. Caffeine: Caffeine is a stimulant that can contribute to silent reflux. If you can't give up caffeine, try to limit your intake to no more than one or two cups of coffee or tea per day. Alcohol: Alcohol is a common trigger for silent reflux. If you enjoy alcohol, limit your intake to no more than one or two drinks per day. Carbonated drinks: Carbonated drinks are a common trigger food for people with silent reflux. If you enjoy carbonated drinks, try to limit your intake to no more than one or two per day. While trigger foods can vary from person to person, these are some of the most common foods that can make silent reflux worse. By avoiding these foods, you can help to control your silent reflux and get your symptoms under control.

Can you feel sick with silent reflux?

The condition known as silent reflux can cause a number of different symptoms, not all of them necessarily involving vomiting or nausea. It is possible to feel sick as a result of silent reflux, but there are many other potential symptoms as well. Silent reflux, also known as laryngopharyngeal reflux (LPR) or extraesophageal reflux disease (EERD), is a condition in which stomach contents and acid back up into the throat and mouth. The main difference between silent reflux and other types of reflux is that silent reflux does not necessarily cause the typical symptoms associated with reflux, such as heartburn. Silent reflux can, however, still lead to damage of the esophagus and other complications. There are a number of different symptoms that can be associated with silent reflux, and not all patients will experience all of them. Some of the more common symptoms include: -throat clearing -coughing -hoarseness -a sensation of a lump in the throat -difficulty swallowing -a sour taste in the mouth -belching -burping -nausea silent reflux can also cause coughing and wheezing in children, and can make asthmatic symptoms worse. If you are experiencing any of these symptoms, it is important to see a doctor to rule out other potential causes and to get a proper diagnosis. Silent reflux can often be managed with lifestyle changes and medication, but it is important to get a proper diagnosis and treatment plan to minimize the risk of complications.

Can anxiety cause silent reflux?

There are many possible causes of acid reflux, and one of them is anxiety. Anxiety can cause a variety of physical symptoms, including chest pain, rapid heartbeat, and difficulty breathing. These symptoms can make it hard to swallow, and can also lead to Silent Reflux. Silent Reflux, also called laryngopharyngeal reflux (LPR), is when stomach acids flow back up into the throat and voice box. This can cause a number of symptoms, including hoarseness, throat clearing, coughing, and difficulty swallowing. Silent Reflux can be particularly frustrating because the symptoms can be hard to pin down. Anxiety is often a culprit in Silent Reflux because it can lead to a number of the physical symptoms that can make it difficult to swallow. When you're anxious, your body goes into fight-or-flight mode. This triggers a number of changes, including an increase in heart rate and a tightening of the muscles in your throat. The symptoms of Silent Reflux can be made worse by stress and anxiety. This is because when you're anxious, your body produces more stomach acid. This increase in stomach acid can lead to heartburn and other symptoms of acid reflux. If you think anxiety may be causing your Silent Reflux, there are a few things you can do to help. First, try to reduce the amount of stress in your life. This may mean taking some time for yourself, setting aside time for relaxation, or finding a hobby that you enjoy. You can also try some home remedies for Silent Reflux, such as avoiding trigger foods, elevating your head while you sleep, and not eating close to bedtime. If these home remedies don't help, you may need to see a doctor. Your doctor can help you find a treatment plan that will work for you. This may include changes to your diet, medication, or lifestyle. If you're struggling with Silent Reflux, don't suffer in silence. Talk to your doctor and find a treatment plan that will help you find relief.

Can stress cause silent reflux?

It is not uncommon for people to experience acid reflux, also known as heartburn, on occasion. However, for some people, this may be a more frequent occurrence. When acid reflux happens frequently, it is called gastroesophageal reflux disease (GERD). While there are many possible causes of GERD, stress may be a factor. There are a few ways that stress could contribute to GERD. First, stress can lead to habits that can trigger GERD, such as smoking and drinking alcohol. second, stress can cause changes in the way the digestive system works, which can lead to GERD. And finally, stress can make it difficult to manage other conditions that may contribute to GERD, such as obesity. While there is no definitive proof that stress causes GERD, many experts believe that it can be a contributing factor. If you are suffering from GERD, it may be important to focus on reducing stress in your life. This may include making lifestyle changes, such as quitting smoking and reducing alcohol consumption. You may also want to try stress-reducing techniques, such as meditation, relaxation, and yoga.

Can probiotics help silent acid reflux?

Silent acid reflux is a condition in which stomach acid flows back up into the esophagus (the tube that carries food from the mouth to the stomach), but does not create the "heartburn" sensation that is associated with traditional acid reflux. This condition can occur at any age, but is most commonly seen in infants and young children. There are a few different ways that probiotics can help silent acid reflux. First, probiotics can help to increase the acidity of the stomach. This may seem counterintuitive, but stomach acid is actually a good thing. Stomach acid helps to break down food and kill harmful bacteria. The problem with silent acid reflux is that the stomach acid is flowing back up into the esophagus, where it can cause inflammation and damage. By increasing the acidity of the stomach, probiotics can help to prevent the acid from flowing back up into the esophagus. Probiotics can also help to improve the function of the lower esophageal sphincter (LES). The LES is a muscle that separates the stomach from the esophagus. When the LES is functioning properly, it acts as a one-way valve, allowing food and liquid to pass into the stomach, but preventing stomach contents from flowing back up into the esophagus. However, in people with silent acid reflux, the LES is either not functioning properly, or is weakened. This can allow stomach acid to flow back up into the esophagus, causing symptoms like heartburn. There is some evidence to suggest that probiotics can help to improve the function of the LES, and thus help to reduce the symptoms of silent acid reflux.

Probiotics can also help to reduce inflammation in the esophagus, which can also help to reduce the symptoms of silent acid reflux. If you think you may be suffering from silent acid reflux, talk to your doctor. Silent acid reflux is often treated with the same medications used to treat traditional acid reflux, including antacids, proton pump inhibitors, and H2 blockers. In some cases, surgery may be necessary to correct the underlying problem.

Acid reflux is a condition in which acid from the stomach rises up into the esophagus, causing heartburn and other symptoms. Many people experience acid reflux from time to time, but it can become a chronic problem if it happens more than twice a week. There are a number of ways to treat acid reflux, and lifestyle changes can often help to reduce its occurrence.

Does magnesium help with silent reflux?

There are many possible causes of silent reflux, and magnesium deficiency is one of them. However, there is no definitive evidence that magnesium supplements are effective in treating silent reflux. Magnesium is a mineral that is essential for many bodily functions, including muscle contraction, nerve function, and blood sugar control. It is also involved in the production of DNA and RNA. Magnesium deficiency can lead to various health problems, such as migraines, insomnia, and fatigue. Silent reflux is a condition in which stomach acid flows back up into the esophagus, causing symptoms such as heartburn, indigestion, and a sour taste in the mouth. Silent reflux can be difficult to diagnose because it often occurs without the classic symptoms of heartburn and indigestion. There is some evidence that magnesium deficiency may be a contributing factor to silent reflux. In one study, magnesium supplementation was found to reduce the symptoms of silent reflux. However, this study was small and more research is needed to confirm the findings. Magnesium supplements are generally considered safe, but they can cause side effects such as diarrhea and bloating. If you are considering taking magnesium supplements, talk to your doctor first to see if they are right for you.

Why do I have LPR all of a sudden?

LPR, or laryngopharyngeal reflux, is a condition in which stomach acid and other digestive fluids back up into the larynx, or voice box, and the pharynx, or throat. LPR can occur when the lower esophageal sphincter (LES), which is a ring of muscle that separates the esophagus from the stomach, doesn't close properly. There are a number of reasons why someone might suddenly develop LPR. One possibility is that they've developed GERD, or gastroesophageal reflux disease. GERD is a more serious condition that occurs when stomach acid flows back up into the esophagus, the tube that carries food from the mouth to the stomach. People withGERD often experience heartburn, a burning sensation in the chest. Another possibility is that the person has a hiatal hernia. A hiatal hernia occurs when the upper part of the stomach protrudes through an opening in the diaphragm, the muscle that separates the chest from the abdomen. This can weaken the LES and allow stomach acid to flow back up into the esophagus. Certain lifestyle choices can also lead to LPR, such as smoking, being overweight, or eating spicy, fatty, or acidic foods. stress can also play a role, as it can lead to tightness in the throat and contribute to a person's overall anxiety. If you suddenly find yourself dealing with the symptoms of LPR, it's important to see a doctor. LPR can be uncomfortable and even painful, and it can also lead to other health problems, such as ulcers, vocal cord damage, and asthma. Treatment will likely involve making lifestyle changes, such as eating a healthier diet, quitting smoking, and reducing stress. Medications may also be prescribed to help reduce stomach acid production or prevent acid reflux.

Do you burp a lot with silent reflux?

There are a few things that could be going on if you're burping a lot with silent reflux. One is that you could be swallowing a lot of air. When you have silent reflux, stomach acid can come up into your throat and mouth. If you're Swallowing a lot of air, that can increase the amount of acid that comes up. Another possibility is that you have a hiatal hernia. A hiatal hernia is when part of your stomach protrudes through your diaphragm into your chest. This can cause Silent reflux because it weakens the barrier that prevents stomach acid from coming up. If you have a hiatal hernia, you may need surgery to fix it. Speak to your doctor to see if a hiatal hernia could be the cause of your burping.

What is similar to silent reflux?

Acid reflux is a condition in which stomach acid flows back up into the esophagus, causing a burning sensation in the chest or throat. Silent reflux is a similar condition, but the main difference is that there are no symptoms associated with silent reflux. This means that people with silent reflux may not even know that they have it. There are a few things that can contribute to silent reflux. One is eating large meals or lying down right after eating. This can cause the stomach acid to flow back up into the esophagus. Another is being overweight or obese. This is because extra weight can put pressure on the stomach, which can cause the acid to flow back up. There are a few things that you can do to help manage or prevent silent reflux. One is to eat smaller meals and not lie down right after eating. Another is to lose weight if you are overweight or obese. You can also sleep with your head elevated to help prevent the acid from flowing back up. If you think that you may have silent reflux, it is important to talk to your doctor. They will be able to give you a more specific diagnosis and talk to you about treatment options.

Can neck problems cause acid reflux?

While neck problems do not seem like they would be related to something like acid reflux, there is actually a connection between the two. It is not fully understood how the two are linked, but there are some theories. One theory is that neck problems can lead to acid reflux because of the way they can change the alignment of the spine. This can then put pressure on the stomach, which can lead to acid reflux. Another theory is that neck problems can cause acid reflux because of the way they can impact the nervous system. This can lead to a change in the way the stomach works, which can then lead to acid reflux. There is no one definitive answer as to how neck problems and acid reflux are connected. However, there are some theories that suggest that there is a link between the two. If you are struggling with acid reflux, it may be worth talking to your doctor about whether or not your neck could be contributing to the problem.

What does GERD anxiety feel like?

Anxiety is a feeling of worry, nervousness, or unease, typically about an imminent event or something with an uncertain outcome. People with anxiety disorders often have recurring intrusive thoughts or concerns. They may avoid certain situations out of worry. They may also have physical symptoms such as sweating, heart palpitations, and dizziness. GERD, or gastroesophageal reflux disease, is a condition where acid from the stomach flows back up into the esophagus. This can cause heartburn, chest pain, and difficulty swallowing. Anxiety can make these symptoms worse. People with anxiety and GERD may be constantly worried about their symptoms. They may feel like they are going to have a heart attack or that they are choking. This can cause a great deal of stress and anxiety. Treatment for GERD can help reduce these symptoms.

How long does LPR take to heal?

LPR, or laryngopharyngeal reflux, is a condition that occurs when stomach acid backs up into the larynx and pharynx, the voice box and throat. LPR is similar to GERD, or gastroesophageal reflux disease, which is a more well-known condition that affects the esophagus, or food pipe. However, LPR is less well-known and often goes undiagnosed because its symptoms are more subtle. The most common symptom of LPR is hoarseness, or a change in the quality of your voice. You may also experience a sensation of burning or tickling in the back of your throat, difficulty swallowing, or a feeling of a lump in your throat. These symptoms can occur at any time, but are more likely to happen after eating or drinking. They may also be worse when you lie down or bend over. LPR is caused by stomach acid that flows backward up into the esophagus and throat. This happens when the valve between the stomach and esophagus, known as the lower esophageal sphincter, or LES, doesn't close properly. The LES is a muscle that opens to allow food and liquid into the stomach, and then closes to keep the contents of the stomach in the stomach. When the LES doesn't close properly, stomach acid can flow backward into the esophagus. There are a number of things that can contribute to the LES not closing properly, including obesity, pregnancy, and smoking. Some medications, such as antacids, can also contribute to LES dysfunction. Most people with LPR don't need treatment, as the condition often improves on its own. However, some people may need medication to reduce the amount of stomach acid. If you think you may have LPR, it's important to see your doctor for a diagnosis. LPR can sometimes be a sign of a more serious condition, such as gastroesophageal junction cancer. Your doctor will likely start with a physical exam and ask about your symptoms. They may also order tests, such as a pH test, to measure the level of acid in your esophagus. Treatment for LPR usually involves lifestyle changes and medications. Some of the lifestyle changes that may help include: - avoiding trigger foods and beverages, such as acidic, spicy, or fatty foods - avoiding tobacco - avoiding caffeine - losing weight - avoiding lying down within three hours of eating - sleeping with the head of your bed elevated Medications that may be used to treat LPR include: - antacids - H2 blockers, which reduce stomach acid production - proton pump inhibitors, which reduce stomach acid production In some cases, surgery may be necessary to tighten the LES. This surgery is typically

While the causes of acid reflux are many and varied, there are a few simple things you can do to help prevent it. Avoiding foods that trigger your reflux, eating smaller meals, and avoiding eating late at night can all help. In addition, losing weight if you are overweight, and avoiding tobacco and alcohol can also help reduce your risk of acid reflux.

Chapter Twenty-Four

What exercise strengthens the esophageal sphincter?

The esophageal sphincter is a ring of muscle that separates the esophagus from the stomach. When this muscle is weak, stomach acids can back up into the esophagus, causing heartburn and other symptoms of acid reflux. There are a few different exercises that can help to strengthen the esophageal sphincter. One is the Valsalva maneuver, which is done by exhaling forcefully with the mouth and nose closed. This can help to increase the pressure in the abdomen and tighten the esophageal sphincter. Another exercise that can help is the swallow close. This is done by taking a small sip of water and then swallowing it without inhaling. This helps to train the muscles around the esophagus to close more tightly. Finally, hiatus hernia exercises can also be helpful. These are exercises that help to push the stomach back up into its proper place. This can help to take the pressure off of the esophageal sphincter and prevent acids from backing up. All of these exercises can help to strengthen the esophageal sphincter and reduce the symptoms of acid reflux. It is important to talk to a doctor before starting any new exercise program, especially if you have any medical conditions.

What happens if LPR goes untreated?

Acid reflux, also known as gastroesophageal reflux disease (GERD), is a condition where acids in the stomach leak back up into the esophagus. GERD can cause a burning sensation in the chest, known as heartburn, as well as a sour, acidic taste in the mouth. Left untreated, GERD can lead to a number of complications, such as: - Barrett's esophagus: a condition where the lining of the esophagus is damaged, increasing the risk of esophageal cancer - Esophagitis: an inflammation of the esophagus - Strictures: a narrowing of the esophagus - Ulcers: sores that form in the esophagus If you think you may be suffering from GERD, it's important to see your doctor so that you can get started on treatment. Left untreated, GERD can have serious consequences.

What are the symptoms of laryngopharyngeal reflux?

Laryngopharyngeal reflux (LPR) is a type of acid reflux where stomach acid flows backward up into the throat and voice box. This can lead to a number of bothersome or even painful symptoms, including: Heartburn: A burning sensation in the chest that is often worse when lying down or bending over. Regurgitation: A feeling of acid backflow that may reach the back of the throat or be felt as heartburn. Dysphagia: difficulty swallowing Globus sensation: the feeling of a lump in the throat that does not go away Cough Hoarseness Sore throat These symptoms may worsen when eating, and can sometimes lead to aspiration pneumonia. LPR is often caused by a weakened or relaxed lower esophageal sphincter (LES). The LES is a ring of muscle that acts like a valve between the stomach and the esophagus. When this muscle is weakened or relaxes, stomach acid can flow backward into the esophagus. LPR can also be caused by other conditions, such as: Pregnancy Obesity Hiatal hernia Smoking Drug use The best way to prevent LPR is to avoid trigger foods and beverages, eat small meals, and avoid eating close to bedtime. Weight loss, elevating the head of the bed, and avoiding reclining for 3 hours after eating can also help. If these lifestyle changes do not improve symptoms, your doctor may prescribe medications to reduce stomach acid production.

Does laryngopharyngeal reflux ever go away?

Laryngopharyngeal reflux (LPR) is a condition in which stomach contents and acid flow back up from the stomach into the esophagus and throat, often causing symptoms such as heartburn, trouble swallowing, and hoarseness. While LPR is similar to gastroesophageal reflux disease (GERD), the two conditions are quite different. GERD is a much more common condition that occurs when stomach acid flows back up into the esophagus. LPR is less common but can be more serious, as the acid can flow all the way up to the larynx (voice box) and even the lungs, causing difficulty breathing. The good news is that, for most people, LPR can be managed and controlled with lifestyle changes and medication. Some people find that making changes to their diet, such as avoiding acidic foods, spicy foods, and fatty foods, helps to reduce their symptoms. Others may need to avoid eating late at night or eating large meals. In addition, over-the-counter and prescription medications can be used to control the symptoms of LPR. Antacids, such as Maalox and Tums, can help to neutralize stomach acid. H2 blockers, such as Zantac and Pepcid, can help to reduce the amount of acid produced by the stomach. And proton pump inhibitors, such as Nexium and Prilosec, can help to block the acid production altogether. For some people, making lifestyle changes and taking medication may not be enough to control their symptoms. In these cases, surgery may be recommended. There are a few different types of surgery that can be used to treat LPR, and the best option for each individual will depend on the severity of their condition and their overall health. The good news is that, for most people, LPR is a treatable condition. With lifestyle changes and medication, most people are able to control their symptoms and live relatively normal lives.

How long does it take to heal laryngopharyngeal reflux?

Laryngopharyngeal reflux (LPR) is a type of digestive disorder that affects the throat and voice box. The main symptom of LPR is heartburn, which is a burning sensation in the chest. Other symptoms include hoarseness, difficulty swallowing, and a feeling of a lump in the throat. LPR is caused by a combination of stomach acid and digestive enzymes that reflux back up the esophagus and into the throat. The good news is that LPR is usually a curable condition. Most people can heal their LPR with a combination of lifestyle changes and medication. The first step is to identify and avoid the foods and beverages that trigger your symptoms. Common triggers include citrus fruits, tomatoes, chocolate, fatty foods, coffee, and alcohol. You should also avoid eating large meals, lying down after eating, and eating late at night. In addition to making dietary changes, you will also need to take medication to reduce stomach acid and help heal your esophagus. The most common type of medication is a proton pump inhibitor (PPI), which blocks the production of stomach acid. PPIs are available over-the-counter or by prescription. Other medication options include antacids, histamine-2 blockers, and prokinetics. Most people with LPR will see a noticeable improvement in their symptoms within a few weeks of starting treatment. However, it can take up to several months for the symptoms to go away completely. If your symptoms do not improve after four to eight weeks of treatment, you may need to see a gastroenterologist for further evaluation.

What is the fastest way to cure LPR?

LPR, or acid reflux, is a condition in which stomach acid backs up into the throat. This can cause a burning sensation in the throat, as well as a sour or bitter taste in the mouth. LPR is often referred to as silent reflux because it can occur without any noticeable symptoms. There are a few different ways to treat LPR, but the fastest way to cure it is to treat the underlying cause. The most common cause of LPR is GERD, or gastroesophageal reflux disease. GERD is a condition in which the lower esophageal sphincter (LES) does not close properly, allowing stomach acid to back up into the esophagus. treatments include lifestyle changes, such as avoiding spicy or fatty foods, eating smaller meals, and not eating late at night. There are also a number of medications that can be used to treat GERD and LPR, such as antacids, H2 blockers, and proton pump inhibitors (PPIs). Surgery is also an option for people who do not respond to other treatments. If you think you may be suffering from LPR, it is important to see your doctor for a diagnosis. LPR is a treatable condition, but it is important to catch it early so that it does not cause any damage to the esophagus.

Why is LPR so hard to treat?

When most people think of acid reflux, they think of the occasional heartburn that comes after eating too much spicy food. However, there is a more serious form of acid reflux known as laryngopharyngeal reflux (LPR). LPR is a condition in which stomach acid and other digestive juices rise up into the throat and mouth. It can cause a variety of symptoms, including heartburn, hoarseness, difficulty swallowing, and a sensation of a lump in the throat. LPR is often referred to as silent reflux because many of its symptoms are silent, or do not produce the typical "heartburn" sensation. This makes LPR much harder to diagnose than GERD (gastroesophageal reflux disease), which is the more well-known form of acid reflux. Furthermore, LPR can occur without any obvious symptoms at all. This makes it even more difficult to diagnose and treat. There are a few theories as to why LPR is so hard to treat. One theory is that LPR is caused by a dysfunction of the lower esophageal sphincter (LES). The LES is a ring of muscle that separates the stomach from the esophagus. Normally, the LES closes tightly to prevent stomach contents from flowing back up into the esophagus. However, in people with LPR, the LES may not close properly, allowing stomach acid and other digestive juices to flow back up into the throat. Another theory is that LPR is caused by a weakened or damaged mucosal barrier. The mucosal barrier is a layer of mucus that lines the digestive tract and helps to protect it from stomach acid. In people with LPR, the mucosal barrier may be weakened or damaged, allowing stomach acid to come into contact with the sensitive tissues of the throat and mouth. There is no one-size-fits-all treatment for LPR. Many people find that a combination of lifestyle changes and medication is necessary to control their symptoms. Lifestyle changes may include avoiding triggers (such as spicy food or coffee), eating smaller meals, and not eating close to bedtime. Medications that may be used to treat LPR include antacids, H2 blockers, and proton pump inhibitors (PPIs). If you think you may have LPR, it is important to see a doctor for an accurate diagnosis. LPR is a serious condition that can lead to serious complications if left untreated. With proper treatment, however, many people with LPR are able to find relief from their symptoms and live normal, healthy lives.

Acid reflux is a condition that affects many people. It can be caused by a number of factors, such as diet, lifestyle, and medications. While it is not a serious condition, it can be uncomfortable and even painful for some people. There are a number of ways to treat acid reflux, such as changes in diet, lifestyle, and medications.

What makes LPR worse?

Acid reflux, also known as gastroesophageal reflux disease (GERD), is a common condition that affects millions of people worldwide.GERD occurs when stomach acid or other digestive fluids back up into the esophagus, the tube that connects the mouth to the stomach. There are a number of factors that can contribute to symptoms of GERD and make the condition worse. Some of the more common causes include: -Overeating or eating large meals -Eating certain foods that trigger reflux, such as fatty foods, spicy foods, caffeine, chocolate, and citrus fruits -Drinking carbonated beverages or alcohol -Smoking -Being overweight or obese -Wearing tight-fitting clothing that puts pressure on the abdomen -Eating close to bedtime -Sleeping on your back or stomach -Pregnancy -Certain medical conditions, such as hiatal hernia, diabetes, and GERD While there are many potential causes of GERD, modifying your lifestyle and diet is often the best place to start when trying to reduce symptoms. Avoiding trigger foods, eating smaller meals, losing weight if necessary, and not eating close to bedtime can often make a big difference. If lifestyle changes don't seem to help, your doctor may prescribe medication to treat GERD. There are a number of different options available, and the best one for you will depend on your individual situation. While GERD can be a nuisance, it's important to remember that it is a very treatable condition. Making some simple lifestyle changes can often provide significant relief. If not, there are many effective medications available that can help you find relief and get back to enjoying your life.

What foods to avoid with LPR?

Chronic reflux, including silent reflux, is a common problem. The symptoms are the same as those of GERD, but they don't respond as well to treatment. Some research suggests that people with silent reflux may be more sensitive to certain foods. People with LPR should avoid trigger foods that are known to promote reflux. Common triggers include spicy foods, fatty foods, tomatoes, citrus fruits, garlic, onion, caffeine, and m int.Trigger foods will vary from person to person, so it is important to pay attention to your own body and what makes your symptoms worse. Eating large meals and eating before bed are both activities that can trigger reflux. Eating smaller meals more frequently throughout the day can help reduce symptoms. It is also important to avoid eating for at least two hours before bedtime. Maintaining a healthy weight is important for people with

LPR. Excess weight can put pressure on the stomach, which can make reflux more likely. Losing weight if you are overweight or obese can help reduce symptoms. People with LPR should avoid tobacco use. Cigarette smoking can weaken the lower esophageal sphincter and increase the risk of reflux. Quitting smoking is the most effective way to reduce the risk of LPR. Avoiding trigger foods and eating smaller meals more frequently throughout the day can help reduce symptoms of LPR. Maintaining a healthy weight is also important. People with LPR should avoid tobacco use. Quitting smoking is the best way to reduce the risk of silent reflux.

How do you heal a LPR throat?

Acid reflux, or gastroesophageal reflux disease (GERD), is a condition in which stomach acids rise up into the esophagus. This can cause a burning sensation in the chest or throat, known as heartburn. GERD is a chronic condition, and it is important to find a way to manage it long-term. There are a few different ways to heal a LPR throat. First, it is important to identify any trigger foods and avoid them. Common trigger foods include caffeine, alcohol, fatty foods, spicy foods, and citrus fruits. It is also important to eat smaller meals more often, and to avoid eating late at night. In addition to dietary changes, there are a number of lifestyle changes that can help to heal a LPR throat. Avoiding tobacco products and wearing loose-fitting clothing can help to prevent symptoms. It is also important to elevate the head of the bed by six to eight inches, to keep stomach acids from rising up into the esophagus while sleeping. There are also a number of medications that can help to heal a LPR throat. Over-the-counter antacids can be taken to neutralize stomach acids. There are also medications called proton pump inhibitors (PPIs), which work to reduce the amount of acid produced by the stomach. PPIs are available both over-the-counter and by prescription. If lifestyle changes and medications do not adequately relieve symptoms, surgery may be an option. If you suffer from LPR, it is important to work with your doctor to find a treatment plan that works for you. With the right treatment, you can heal your LPR throat and get back to enjoying your life.

Can LPR damage lungs?

Laryngopharyngeal reflux (LPR), also known as extraesophageal reflux disease (EERD), silent reflux, and supra-esophageal reflux, is a form of gastroesophageal reflux disease (GERD). LPR can occur during the day or night, even when a person is not eating. The primary symptom of LPR is heartburn, which is also known as acid reflux. However, unlike GERD, heartburn caused by LPR is often not accompanied by a burning sensation in the chest. Other common symptoms of LPR include: - A sensation of a lump in the throat - A feeling of mucus or phlegm in the back of the throat - A chronic cough - A hoarse voice LPR is a serious condition that can lead to a number of complications, including damage to the lungs. In some cases, LPR can cause aspiration pneumonia, which is a type of pneumonia that occurs when liquids, food, or stomach acid is aspirated (inhaled) into the lungs. Aspiration pneumonia is a serious condition that can be life-threatening. If you think you may have LPR, it is important to see a doctor so that you can be properly diagnosed and treated.

What is considered severe LPR?

LPR, or acid reflux, is a common condition in which stomach acid rises up into the throat. While occasional acid reflux is normal, severe LPR can be a potentially serious condition. Severe LPR is often characterized by symptoms that occur more than twice a week. These symptoms may include heartburn, a sour taste in the mouth, difficulty swallowing, and a hoarse voice. Severe LPR can also lead to GERD, or gastroesophageal reflux disease. GERD is a more serious condition that can cause serious health complications. Treatment for severe LPR usually involves a combination of lifestyle changes and medication. Making lifestyle changes, such as avoiding trigger foods and eating smaller meals, can help to reduce the symptoms of LPR. Medications, such as antacids and proton pump inhibitors, can also be effective in treating severe LPR. If you are experiencing symptoms of severe LPR, it is important to see a doctor so that you can receive treatment. Severe LPR is a treatable condition, but left untreated, it can lead to serious health complications.

Does Gaviscon help laryngopharyngeal reflux?

There is no one-size-fits-all answer to the question of whether or not Gaviscon can help with laryngopharyngeal reflux (LPR). It may help some people while not helping others. The reason for this is that the causes of LPR are varied, and so are the effects of Gaviscon. Gaviscon is a medication that is used to treat heartburn and gastroesophageal reflux disease (GERD). It works by increasing the amount of time that stomach acid stays in the stomach, and by forming a barrier that prevents stomach acid from moving up into the esophagus. Gaviscon comes in liquid and tablet form, and is taken after meals and at bedtime. LPR is a condition in which stomach acid refluxes up into the throat. LPR can cause a number of symptoms, including throat soreness, hoarseness, cough, and trouble swallowing. LPR is often diagnosed in people who have GERD, although it can occur in people who do not have GERD. The cause of LPR is not always clear. It is thought to be related to a combination of factors, including a weakened esophageal sphincter, a hiatal hernia, and certain lifestyle factors such as eating large meals, lying down after eating, and eating spicy or acidic foods. Management of LPR often focuses on lifestyle changes, such as avoiding trigger foods and beverages, eating smaller meals, and avoiding lying down for at least three hours after eating. Some people also find that elevation of the head of their bed can help to reduce symptoms. In some cases, medications may be necessary to control symptoms. Medications that are commonly used to treat LPR include proton pump inhibitors (PPIs) and antacids. PPIs work by blocking the production of stomach acid. Antacids work by neutralizing stomach acid. Gaviscon is an antacid. There is no clear evidence that Gaviscon is effective in treating LPR. However, some people find that it helps to reduce their symptoms. Gaviscon is generally considered to be safe, and side effects are rare. If you are considering taking Gaviscon for LPR, it is important to speak to your doctor first to discuss whether it is right for you.

How do you get Laryngopharyngeal reflux?

Laryngopharyngeal reflux (LPR) is a condition in which stomach acid and other contents of the stomach flow back up into the larynx (voice box) and pharynx (throat). LPR is also known as silent reflux because it often does not cause any symptoms. LPR occurs when the lower esophageal sphincter (LES) does not close properly and stomach contents flow back up into the esophagus. The LES is a ring of muscle that separates the esophagus from the stomach. When the LES relaxes, stomach contents can flow back up into the esophagus. This is called reflux. The LES is supposed to close tightly after food has passed through it. However, sometimes the LES relaxes or weakens when it should stay shut. This allows stomach acid and other contents to leak back up into the esophagus. There are several factors that can contribute to the LES relaxing or weakening, including: -Eating large meals -Eating certain foods, such as spicy foods, fatty foods, chocolate, caffeine, or mint -Drinking alcohol -Smoking -Being overweight or obese -Pregnancy -Taking certain medications, such as calcium channel blockers, beta blockers, or nitrates LPR can cause a number of symptoms, including: - Heartburn - Chest pain - Difficulty swallowing - Hoarseness - A feeling of a lump in the throat - Sore throat - Cough LPR can be a serious condition if left untreated. Over time, LPR can damage the esophagus and even lead to cancer. If you think you may have LPR, it is important to see a doctor so that you can get treatment. There are a number of different treatments for LPR, including: - Diet changes - Weight loss - Avoiding triggers - Medicines - Surgery

While acid reflux is not usually a serious condition, it can be uncomfortable and inconvenient. There are a few simple lifestyle changes you can make to help relieve your symptoms. Avoiding spicy, fatty, or acidic foods can help, as can avoiding eating late at night or lying down right after eating. If lifestyle changes don't help, your doctor may prescribe medication to treat your acid reflux.

Does probiotics help LPR?

Probiotics are live microorganisms, typically bacteria, that are similar to the ones already present in our gut. More and more research is emerging on the potential health benefits of probiotics, including for acid reflux or laryngopharyngeal reflux (LPR). LPR is when stomach contents and acid back up into the throat and larynx, which can cause symptoms like heartburn, hoarseness, and difficulty swallowing. There are different probiotics available, and they can be found in supplements, foods, and even some topical products. The exact way that probiotics work is still not fully understood, but it is thought that they may help to improve gut motility and digestion, reduce inflammation, and enhance the barrier function of the gut lining. Probiotics may also help to change the composition of the gut microbiota, which is the community of microorganisms that live in our gut. A recent systematic review and meta-analysis concluded that probiotics may be effective in reducing symptoms of LPR. The study found that probiotics were associated with a significant reduction in heartburn, acid regurgitation, and belching. Probiotics were also associated with a significant reduction in the number of reflux episodes and the duration of reflux episodes. The most commonly used probiotics for LPR are Lactobacillus and Bifidobacterium. These are the same types of probiotics that are often found in yogurt and other fermented foods. Probiotics are generally considered to be safe, but as with any supplement, it is always best to speak with a healthcare professional before starting any new supplement, especially if you have a medical condition. If you are considering taking probiotics for LPR, it is important to choose a quality product. Look for a product that contains a minimum of 1 billion CFUs (colony forming units) per serving, and that has been shown to be effective in clinical studies. It is also important to take probiotics consistently, for at least 4-8 weeks, in order to see results.

When should I be concerned about LPR?

Laryngopharyngeal reflux (LPR) is a condition that occurs when stomach contents and acid back up from the stomach into the voice box, or throat. LPR can occur during the day or night, even if a person has not eaten recently. The most common symptoms of LPR are hoarseness, a chronic cough, wheezing, and difficulty swallowing. LPR can also cause heartburn, a sour taste in the mouth, or a burning sensation in the chest. These symptoms usually occur after eating or drinking, or when lying down. If you experience any of these symptoms, you should see your doctor to rule out other causes, such as GERD or a viral infection. If LPR is diagnosed, your doctor may recommend lifestyle changes and medications to treat the condition.

What happens if you dont treat LPR?

If you suffer from acid reflux and don't treat it, the acidic stomach contents will reflux back up the esophagus. This can cause symptoms such as heartburn, chest pain, and a sour taste in your mouth. untreated acid reflux may also contribute to the development of Barrett's esophagus, a serious condition that can lead to cancer. If you think you may have acid reflux, talk to your doctor.

Is yogurt good for LPR reflux?

There isn't a one-size-fits-all answer to this question, as the effectiveness of yogurt as a treatment for acid reflux will vary from person to person. However, yogurt is generally considered to be a health food, and so it is unlikely to do any harm if you try it as a treatment for your acid reflux. Acid reflux, also known as gastroesophageal reflux disease (GERD), is a condition where stomach acid rises up into the esophagus. This can cause heartburn, chest pain, and damage to the esophagus. GERD is a chronic condition, and it can be difficult to treat. There are many possible treatments for GERD, and yogurt is one of them. yogurt is thought to be a good treatment for acid reflux because it is a probiotic. Probiotics are live bacteria and yeasts that are good for your health, and they are often found in fermented foods like yogurt. Probiotics can help improve gut health, and this is thought to be helpful for people with GERD. Yogurt is also a good source of calcium. Calcium is thought to help reduce the amount of acid produced by the stomach. This may help to reduce the symptoms of acid reflux. If you are considering trying yogurt as a treatment for your acid reflux, it is important to choose a yogurt that is plain and unsweetened. Sweetened yogurts may contain sugar, which can trigger acid reflux. It is also a good idea to choose a yogurt that is full-fat, as this may be more soothing to the digestive system.

Do antihistamines help LPR?

The answer to this question is unfortunately not as straightforward as one might hope. While there are anecdotal reports that antihistamines have helped alleviate symptoms of laryngopharyngeal reflux (LPR), the scientific evidence to support this is lacking. One small study looked at the effect of cetirizine (a common antihistamine) in LPR patients and found that it helped reduce symptoms such as heartburn and nausea. However, this study was not well designed and thus its results should be interpreted with caution. There are also a few case reports of people with LPR who found relief from their symptoms after taking antihistamines. However, it is difficult to know if the antihistamines were truly responsible for the improvement, or if it was simply a coincidence. Overall, there is currently not enough evidence to recommend the use of antihistamines for the treatment of LPR. If you are experiencing symptoms of LPR, it is best to speak with your doctor to find an evidence-based treatment that is right for you.

What supplements are good for LPR?

Acid reflux is a condition in which stomach acid backs up into the esophagus, causing heartburn and other symptoms. There are a number of supplements that may help to relieve the symptoms of LPR, including: - Antacids: These work to neutralize stomach acid, helping to relieve heartburn and other symptoms. - Alginates: These work by forming a barrier between the stomach acid and the esophagus, helping to prevent acid reflux. - H2-receptor blockers: These work by reducing the production of stomach acid, helping to prevent acid reflux. - Proton pump inhibitors: These work by blocking the action of stomach acid pumps, helping to reduce the amount of stomach acid and prevent acid reflux.

How do you treat LPR naturally?

Acid reflux, also known as GERD, is a condition where the acidic contents of the stomach flow back up into the esophagus. This can lead to a burning sensation in the chest and throat, as well as other symptoms like difficulty swallowing, bad breath, and a sour taste in the mouth. There are a number of things you can do to treat LPR naturally. One of the most important is to avoid trigger foods and beverages. Common trigger foods include coffee, alcohol, spicy foods, fatty foods, and chocolate. You may also want to avoid eating late at night or lying down immediately after eating. Another important step in treating LPR naturally is to improve your gut health. This can be done by consuming probiotic-rich foods like yogurt, sauerkraut, and kimchi, as well as taking a probiotic supplement. Additionally, you can promote gut health by eating plenty of fiber-rich foods and avoiding foods that promote inflammation. Finally, it's important to manage stress levels. Stress can contribute to LPR by increasing acid production and relaxing the lower esophageal sphincter. To reduce stress, you may want to try relaxation techniques like yoga, meditation, and deep breathing. By following these natural treatment options, you can improve your symptoms of LPR and promote gut health.

Acid reflux can be a painful and dangerous condition if left untreated. However, with proper treatment and lifestyle changes, it can be managed effectively. If you suspect that you may have acid reflux, be sure to see your doctor for an accurate diagnosis and treatment plan.

Can LPR lead to COPD?

Can LPR lead to COPD? There is some debate as to whether or not LPR can lead to COPD. Some studies suggest that there is a link between the two conditions, while other research suggests that LPR does not increase the risk of developing COPD. LPR stands for laryngopharyngeal reflux. This occurs when stomach acid and other digestive juices flow back up the esophagus and into the throat. LPR can cause a number of symptoms, including heartburn, difficulty swallowing, and a sour taste in the mouth. COPD stands for chronic obstructive pulmonary disease. This is a progressive lung disease that makes it difficult to breathe. COPD is a serious condition that can be fatal. There is some evidence to suggest that LPR can lead to COPD. One study found that LPR was associated with an increased risk of COPD. The study found that people with LPR were more likely to develop COPD than those without LPR. Another study found that LPR was associated with a higher risk of hospitalization for COPD. The study found that people with LPR were more likely to be hospitalized for COPD than those without LPR. Some experts believe that LPR can cause inflammation in the lungs, which may lead to COPD. In addition, LPR can damage the airways, which can also lead to COPD. While there is some evidence to suggest that LPR can lead to COPD, more research is needed to confirm this link. If you have LPR, you should see your doctor to discuss your risk of developing COPD.

Should I see an ENT or gastroenterologist for LPR?

If you have acid reflux, you may wonder if you should see an ENT or gastroenterologist for your condition. While both specialty doctors can treat acid reflux, there are some differences between the two. ENTs, or otolaryngologists, are ear, nose, and throat specialists. They are trained in the surgical and medical treatment of the head and neck, and have expertise in disorders of the ear, nose, throat, and larynx (voice box). Many ENTs also treat allergies and sinus disorders. Gastroenterologists are doctors who specialize in the diagnosis and treatment of disorders of the gastrointestinal tract, which includes the esophagus, stomach, small intestine, large intestine, pancreas, and gallbladder. Gastroenterologists are often able to treat acid reflux with lifestyle changes and medication. In some cases, surgery may be necessary to treat acid reflux. So, should you see an ENT or gastroenterologist for acid reflux? If you have symptoms of acid reflux, such as heartburn, chest pain, or trouble swallowing, you should see a doctor for an evaluation. If you have LPR, you may also have symptoms such as hoarseness, sore throat, or coughing. In general, if you have symptoms that are affecting your quality of life, you should see a doctor for an evaluation.

What is the best antacid for LPR?

Acid reflux, also known as gastroesophageal reflux (GERD), is a condition where stomach acid rises up into the esophagus. This can cause heartburn, chest pain, and regurgitation. There are many over-the-counter (OTC) and prescription medications available to treat acid reflux. Antacids are often the first line of treatment. These drugs work to neutralize the stomach acid. There are many different types and brands of antacids available. Some examples include Tums, Rolaids, Maalox, and Pepto-Bismol. Antacids are usually taken after meals and at bedtime. They can be taken as a liquid, chewable tablet, or capsule. While antacids are effective at relieving symptoms, they do not address the underlying cause of the condition. For that, you will need a stronger medication, such as a proton pump inhibitor (PPI). If you have occasional acid reflux, antacids are a good first-line of treatment. If you have more frequent or severe symptoms, you may need a PPI. Speak with your doctor to determine the best course of treatment for your individual needs.

Will omeprazole cure LPR?

LPR, or acid reflux, is a condition in which stomach acid backs up into the throat. This can cause a burning sensation in the throat and chest, as well as a sour taste in the mouth. Many people with LPR also have difficulty swallowing. Omeprazole is a medication that is used to treat a variety of gastrointestinal disorders. It is a proton-pump inhibitor, which means that it works to reduce the amount of acid produced in the stomach. There is some evidence to suggest that omeprazole may be effective in treating LPR.

A study published in the Journal of Otolaryngology - Head and Neck Surgery found that omeprazole was effective in reducing symptoms in people with LPR. However, it is important to remember that omeprazole is not a cure for LPR. It is a medication that can help to control the symptoms of the condition. If you have LPR, you will likely need to take omeprazole for a long period of time.

How long does omeprazole take to work for LPR?

Omeprazole is a medication that is used to treat Acid Reflux Disorder, also known as GERD. It is a proton pump inhibitor, which means it works by decreasing the amount of acid that is produced by the stomach. For most people, omeprazole takes about 4 to 8 weeks to work. However, some people may experience relief from their symptoms within a few days. If you are taking omeprazole for the first time, it is important to be patient and give the medication a chance to work. If you do not experience any relief after a few weeks, or if your symptoms get worse, be sure to talk to your doctor.

Are bananas good for acid reflux?

There are a lot of old wives tales about what foods are good for acid reflux and what foods are not. Unfortunately, there is not a lot of evidence to support most of these claims. However, there are a few foods that have been shown to be helpful in reducing acid reflux symptoms. One of these foods is bananas. Bananas are a good source of dietary fiber and have been shown to be helpful in reducing acid reflux symptoms. In addition, bananas are low in acidity and can help to neutralize stomach acid. Furthermore, bananas contain pectin, which has been shown to be effective in reducing acid reflux symptoms. It is important to note that there is no one-size-fits-all approach to managing acid reflux. What works for one person may not work for another. However, including bananas as part of a healthy diet is a good place to start.

Are blueberries good for acid reflux?

Acid reflux is a condition in which the contents of the stomach are regurgitated up into the throat. The main symptom of acid reflux is heartburn, which is a burning sensation in the chest. There are various treatments for acid reflux, but one natural remedy is to eat blueberries. This is because blueberries are thought to decrease the amount of acid in the stomach. There is some evidence to support this claim. A study published in the Journal of Gastroenterology found that people who ate blueberries had a decrease in the amount of acid in their stomach. Another study, published in the World Journal of Gastroenterology, found that blueberries may help to protect the stomach from damage caused by acid reflux. So, if you suffer from acid reflux, it may be worth trying to include blueberries in your diet. However, it is always best to speak to a doctor or dietitian first, as they will be able to advise you on the best course of treatment.

Acid reflux is a condition where the contents of the stomach come back up into the esophagus, irritating the lining and causing pain. It is a common problem, affecting up to 20% of Americans. There are many treatments available, both over-the-counter and prescription, that can help to ease the symptoms of acid reflux. If you suffer from acid reflux, talk to your doctor about the best treatment option for you.

What snacks help reflux?

What snacks help reflux? There are a few snacks that can help you manage your acid reflux. First, try to avoid trigger foods that cause your reflux. Common triggers include caffeine, chocolate, fried foods, and spicy foods.

If you're not sure what your triggers are, keep a food diary and take note of what you eat before your reflux flares up. There are also a few specific snacks that can help manage your acid reflux. For example, yogurt can help soothe your stomach by neutralizing stomach acids. Oatmeal is another good option because it absorbs stomach acid. Additionally, ginger has natural anti-inflammatory properties that can help reduce the irritation caused by reflux. If you're looking for a snack that will help you avoid reflux, try to focus on foods that are low in acid and fat. Fresh fruits and vegetables, whole grain breads, and lean protein are all good choices. When in doubt, talk to your doctor or dietitian about which foods are best for you.

What is the root cause of silent reflux?

What is the root cause of silent reflux? While the symptoms of silent reflux are the same as those of gastroesophageal reflux disease (GERD), the two conditions are quite different. Silent reflux, also known as laryngopharyngeal reflux (LPR), is a type of reflux that occurs when stomach acid and other contents of the stomach flow back up into the larynx, or voice box. This backflow of stomach contents can irritate the lining of the voice box, and cause a number of symptoms, including: - Hoarseness - A "lump" in the throat - Trouble swallowing - Sensation of drainage from the back of the nose - Postnasal drip While GERD is a very common condition, affecting as many as 20% of the population, silent reflux is much less common. It is estimated that only 5-7% of the population suffers from LPR. There are a number of possible causes of silent reflux, but the most likely cause is a dysfunction of the lower esophageal sphincter (LES). The LES is a ring of muscle that separates the stomach from the esophagus. Normally, the LES relaxes to allow food and liquids to flow down into the stomach, and then contracts to prevent them from flowing back up. However, in people with silent reflux, the LES does not function properly, and stomach contents are able to back up into the esophagus. There are a number of lifestyle factors that can contribute to the development of silent reflux, including: - Obesity - Pregnancy - Smoking - Eating large meals - Eating certain foods (such as fatty foods, spicy foods, chocolate, coffee, tea, and citrus fruits) - Wearing tight-fitting clothing - Drinking alcohol If you think you may be suffering from silent reflux, it is important to see a doctor, as the condition can be successfully treated.

Is magnesium good for silent reflux?

There are many treatments for silent reflux, and magnesium is one supplement that is sometimes recommended. Magnesium is a mineral that is involved in many functions in the body, including muscle relaxation. Some people believe that magnesium can help to relax the muscles in the esophagus, which may help to reduce symptoms of silent reflux. There is some evidence that magnesium may be effective in treating silent reflux. One study found that magnesium supplements reduced the symptoms of GERD in a group of children. However, this study was small, and more research is needed to confirm the effectiveness of magnesium for silent reflux. magnesium is generally considered to be safe, and side effects are rare. However, magnesium can interact with some medications, so it is important to speak to a doctor before taking magnesium supplements. overall, magnesium is a promising treatment for silent reflux, and it is generally safe and well-tolerated. However, more research is needed to confirm its effectiveness. If you are considering taking magnesium supplements, speak to a doctor first to make sure it is safe for you.

What are five vitamins to stop acid reflux?

There are a few vitamins that have been shown to be effective in minimizing the symptoms of acid reflux. Here are five of them: Vitamin C: This vitamin is a natural acid neutralizer. It can be taken in supplement form or found in foods like citrus fruits, tomatoes, and Brussels sprouts. Vitamin B complex: These vitamins help the body to break down and use proteins and carbohydrates, which can minimize the amount of acid produced in the stomach. They can be found in foods like whole grains, beans, and dark leafy greens. Vitamin D: This vitamin helps to absorb calcium, which can help to reduce the amount of acid in the stomach. It can be found in fortified foods like milk and cereal, as well as in fatty fish like salmon and tuna. Vitamin E: This vitamin has anti-inflammatory properties, which can help to reduce the inflammation caused by acid reflux. It can be found in foods like nuts and seeds, as well as in supplement form. Vitamin A: This vitamin also has anti-inflammatory properties, which can help to reduce the symptoms of acid reflux. It can be found in foods like carrots, sweet potatoes, and dark leafy greens.

What are the 8 symptoms of GERD?

Gastroesophageal reflux disease (GERD) is a condition that causes the contents of your stomach to wash back up into your esophagus, throat, and mouth. This can happen when the opening between your stomach and esophagus weakens or relaxes.GERD can cause heartburn, which is a burning sensation in the middle of your chest. It can also cause other symptoms such as: -coughing -wheezing -chest pain -a bad taste in your mouth -hoarseness -difficulty swallowing If you have any of these symptoms, you should see your doctor. GERD can be treated with over-the-counter medicines and lifestyle changes. GERD is a chronic (long-term) condition. It can occur intermittently or continuously. Intermittent GERD happens when you have episodes of heartburn that are not related to certain triggers. Continuous GERD happens when heartburn occurs more than twice a week. There are a number of lifestyle changes you can make to help relieve your symptoms and stop GERD from getting worse. These include: -quit smoking -lose weight if you are overweight -eat smaller meals -avoid eating late at night -elevate the head of your bed -avoid food and drinks that trigger your symptoms -avoid wearing tight clothing If lifestyle changes do not work, your doctor may prescribe medicine. There are a number of different types of medicine that can help relieve your symptoms. These include: -antacids -H2 blockers -proton pump inhibitors If you have GERD, it is important to see your doctor if your symptoms are not relieved by lifestyle changes or medicine. GERD can lead to serious complications, such as: -esophagitis -esophageal ulcers -Barrett's esophagus -esophageal cancer Esophagitis is inflammation of the lining of the esophagus. This can happen when stomach acid repeatedly washes back up into the esophagus. Esophagitis can cause symptoms such as: -heartburn -chest pain -difficulty swallowing -weight loss Esophageal ulcers are open sores in the lining of the esophagus. They can be caused by GERD or by taking certain medicines, such as aspirin or ibuprofen. Esophageal ulcers can cause symptoms such as: -heartburn -chest pain -difficulty swallowing -weight loss Barrett's esophagus is

How can I get rid of GERD?

There are a few things you can do to get rid of GERD. One is to take antacids. Antacids neutralize stomach acid. Another is to take H2 blockers. H2 blockers reduce the amount of acid your stomach produces. You can also make some lifestyle changes. Avoiding foods that trigger heartburn can help. Common triggers include fried foods, fatty foods, citrus fruits, chocolate, and caffeine. Eating smaller meals more often can also help. And don't lie down right after you eat. Wait at least a couple of hours before you hit the sack. If these lifestyle changes and medications don't help, you may need surgery. One type of surgery is called fundoplication. This procedure strengthens the valve between your stomach and esophagus. This keeps stomach acid from flowing back into your esophagus.

How do you know if you have a GERD?

Acid reflux disease, also known as GERD, is a condition in which the contents of the stomach come back up into the esophagus. This can happen when the lower esophageal sphincter, which is a muscle that separates the stomach from the esophagus, does not close properly. When this happens, the contents of the stomach, which are acidic, can come back up into the esophagus and cause a burning sensation. There are a few different ways that you can tell if you have GERD. One way is if you have a burning sensation in your chest. This is known as heartburn. Heartburn is the most common symptom of GERD. Other symptoms of GERD include: - regurgitation, which is when food or liquid comes back up into the throat - chest pain - trouble swallowing - a hoarse voice If you have any of these symptoms, it is important to see a doctor. They can determine if you have GERD and help you treat it.

Acid reflux is a condition in which stomach acid flows back up into the esophagus, causing heartburn and other symptoms. While it can be annoying and uncomfortable, it is usually not a serious condition. There are a number of things you can do to help relieve your symptoms, such as avoiding trigger foods, eating smaller meals, and elevating your head when you sleep. If you have persistent or severe symptoms, you may need medication or other treatment.

Is GERD that serious?

GERD, or gastroesophageal reflux disease, is a common digestive disorder that afflicts many people. The main symptom of GERD is heartburn, which is a burning sensation in the chest that can extend to the throat and jaw. GERD is caused by a weakness in the lower esophageal sphincter (LES), which is the muscle that separates the stomach from the esophagus.

The LES is responsible for keeping stomach contents from flowing back up into the esophagus. When the LES is weakened, stomach acid and other digestive juices can flow back up into the esophagus, causing heartburn and other symptoms. GERD is a serious condition that can lead to a number of other health problems if left untreated. GERD can damage the esophagus, causing inflammation, ulcers, and bleeding. GERD can also lead to Barrett's esophagus, a condition in which the lining of the esophagus is damaged by stomach acid. Barrett's esophagus can increase the risk of esophageal cancer. If you suffer from heartburn or other symptoms of GERD, it is important to see a doctor. GERD can usually be treated with lifestyle changes and over-the-counter medication. In some cases, surgery may be necessary to repair the LES.

What does a GERD flare up feel like?

A GERD flare up can feel like a burning sensation in your chest or throat. You may also feel like you have food stuck in your throat. Other symptoms can include coughing, belching, and trouble swallowing. Some people may also have a sour taste in their mouth. If you have GERD, you may sometimes wake up in the middle of the night feeling like you are choking or coughing. This can be scary and make it hard to go back to sleep. You may not have all of these symptoms all the time. And some people with GERD may not have any symptoms at all. But when you do have symptoms, they can be bothersome and interfere with your daily life.

What is the fastest way to cure GERD?

There is no one fast way to cure GERD, as the condition is often chronic and requires long-term management. However, there are a few things that can be done to provide relief from symptoms and prevent flare-ups. Avoiding trigger foods, eating smaller meals more often, and elevating the head of the bed are all helpful measures. Additionally, over-the-counter medications like antacids can provide short-term relief. If symptoms are severe, prescription medications may be necessary. In some cases, surgery may be the best option. Ultimately, working with a gastroenterologist to create a customized plan is the best way to manage GERD.

How do you fix GERD naturally?

There are many ways to treat GERD, or acid reflux, naturally. These include lifestyle changes, like eating smaller meals more often and avoiding triggers like spicy foods. Other natural treatments include herbal remedies like licorice root and chamomile, which can help to soothe the gut. Probiotics and digestive enzymes may also be helpful in reducing symptoms. Making some simple changes to your diet can often help to reduce symptoms of GERD. Try to eat smaller meals more often, and avoid trigger foods like spicy dishes, caffeine, and citrus fruits. Fatty and fried foods can also aggravate symptoms, so it's best to avoid these as well. Instead, focus on eating lots of fruits, vegetables, and whole grains. There are also a number of herbal remedies that can be helpful in treating GERD. Licorice root is thought to help heal the lining of the stomach, while chamomile can help to soothe the digestive tract. Probiotics and digestive enzymes may also help to reduce symptoms by aiding in digestion.

Can I cure GERD on my own?

Acid reflux, also known as GERD, is a condition where stomach acid flows back up into the esophagus, causing a burning sensation in the chest or throat. While there is no cure for GERD, there are ways to manage the symptoms and prevent the condition from getting worse. There are a few things you can do at home to manage your GERD symptoms. First, try to avoid trigger foods and beverages. Common trigger foods include fatty or fried foods, spicy foods, citrus fruits, tomatoes, chocolate, mint, and caffeine. If you eat a trigger food, be sure to eat small meals and avoid lying down for at least three hours after eating. Second, you can try to sleep with your head elevated. This will help keep stomach acid from flowing back up into the esophagus. You can prop up your head with pillows or sleep on a wedge pillow. Third, loose-fitting clothing can help to prevent GERD symptoms. Avoid wearing tight belts or clothing that puts pressure on your stomach. Lastly, there are a few lifestyle changes you can make to help prevent GERD. If you are overweight, losing weight can help to reduce symptoms. Avoid smoking and drinking alcohol. Both of these can make GERD symptoms worse. Making these changes may help to reduce your GERD symptoms and prevent the condition from getting worse. However, if you are still experiencing symptoms, it is important to talk to your doctor. They may recommend other treatments, such as medication, to help manage your GERD.

What foods should I avoid if I have GERD?

Some people experience heartburn or acid reflux mild symptoms while others find them very painful and disruptive. There are certain foods that can trigger heartburn or make it worse. It is important to experiment to see what foods trigger your heartburn. Some common foods that may trigger heartburn are: -citrus fruits -tomatoes -chocolate -onions -garlic -peppermint -carbonated beverages -alcohol When you have heartburn, you may feel a burning sensation in your chest or throat. This burning feeling is called acid reflux. Acid reflux occurs when stomach acid backs up into your esophagus. This can happen after you eat, after you bend over, or when you lie down. The symptoms of acid reflux may include: -heartburn -chest pain -difficulty swallowing - Regurgitation of food or sour liquid -burping -hiccups There are a few things you can do to ease the symptoms of acid reflux. -Eat smaller meals more often -Avoidtrigger foods

-Eat slowly -Avoid fatty and fried foods -Avoid beverages that contain caffeine -Avoid alcohol -Quit smoking If you have heartburn more than twice a week, you may have GERD. GERD is a more serious condition that can lead to other problems, such as: -esophagitis -Barrett's esophagus -esophageal ulcers -esophageal stricture If you have GERD, you should see your doctor. They may recommend: -changes in your diet -medication -surgery

What is the main cause of GERD?

The main cause of GERD is a condition called gastroesophageal reflux disease (GERD). This is when the stomach contents, including acid, flow back up into the esophagus. This can happen when the lower esophageal sphincter (LES) muscle weakens or relaxes. The LES is a ring of muscle at the bottom of the esophagus that normally opens to let food in and closes to keep food and acid in the stomach. When this muscle relaxes, acid can flow back up into the esophagus, leading to GERD. There are a number of things that can contribute to the LES muscle weakening or relaxing, including pregnancy, obesity, smoking, and certain medications. diet and lifestyle. There are a number of things that can be done to help reduce the symptoms of GERD, including avoiding trigger foods and drinks, eating smaller meals, and avoiding lying down immediately after eating. Additionally, over-the-counter and prescription medications are available to help treat GERD.

If you are one of the many people who suffer from acid reflux, you know that it can be a painful and disruptive condition. There are many treatments available, but often they do not provide complete relief. Fortunately, there are some simple lifestyle changes that can help. By avoiding triggers, eating smaller meals, and elevating your head during sleep, you can often find significant relief from your symptoms.

What does untreated GERD feel like?

Acid reflux, also known as GERD, can be a painful and disruptive condition. When left untreated, the symptoms of GERD can include: - Heartburn: A burning sensation in the chest that can extend to the throat. - Acid regurgitation: A sour or bitter-tasting fluid that backs up into the throat or mouth. - Dyspepsia: Abdominal pain or discomfort. - Bloating - Belching - Nausea In some cases, GERD can also lead to more serious problems such as esophageal stricture, esophageal ulcers, and Barrett's esophagus. If you think you may be suffering from GERD, it's important to see a doctor for a diagnosis. GERD can usually be treated with lifestyle changes and medication.

How do people get GERD?

There are many different things that can contribute to somebody getting GERD, or gastroesophageal reflux disease. It's often caused by a combination of factors, and sometimes it can be tough to pinpoint exactly what's causing the issue. For starters, GERD can be caused by a malfunctioning valve between the stomach and the esophagus. This valve is supposed to keep the contents of the stomach in, but when it doesn't work properly, those contents can come back up. Another potential cause of GERD is eating certain foods. Spicy, fatty, or acidic foods can all contribute to GERD, as can eating large meals, eating right before bed, or eating late at night. overeating in general can also lead to GERD. Certain medical conditions can also cause, or worsen, GERD. Things like hiatal hernias, pregnancy, and diabetes can all lead to GERD. And GERD is also more common in people who are obese, or who smoke. There are a variety of treatments available for GERD. Many people find that making lifestyle changes, like eating smaller meals, avoiding trigger foods, and not eating right before bed, can help. Others might need to take medication, like antacids, proton pump inhibitors, or H2 blockers. Surgery is also an option for some people with GERD.

Does stress cause GERD?

Acid Reflux and Stress The relationship between acid reflux and stress has been long debated by the medical community. While it is commonly believed that stress can worsen acid reflux symptoms, the evidence to support this claim is not conclusive. There are a number of studies that have looked at the link between stress and acid reflux. One study, published in the journal Psychosomatic Medicine, found that people with acid reflux are more likely to report higher levels of stress than those without the condition. However, the study did not prove that stress causes acid reflux. It is possible that people with acid reflux are more likely to perceive stress than those without the condition. Another study, published in the journal Digestive Diseases and Sciences, found that stress may worsen acid reflux symptoms. The study found that people who were exposed to stress were more likely to have symptoms of acid reflux, such as heartburn and regurgitation. However, the study did not prove that stress causes acid reflux. It is possible that the relationship between stress and acid reflux is bidirectional. It is also worth noting that the studies mentioned above used self-reported measures of stress. This means that the participants were asked about their stress levels after they had already developed acid reflux. It is possible that the participants were more likely to recall times when they were stressed after they had developed acid reflux. This would bias the results of the studies. In conclusion, the evidence to support the claim that stress causes acid reflux is not conclusive. While there are some studies that suggest a link between the two, the evidence is not definitive.

Do people with GERD live long?

It is a common misconception that people with GERD, or Gastroesophageal Reflux Disease, will not live long. This is not the case. In fact, people with GERD can live just as long as people without GERD, provided they take care of themselves and manage their condition. There are a few things that people with GERD can do to help themselves. First, it is important to avoid trigger foods. Common trigger foods include spicy foods, fatty foods, citrus fruits, and caffeine. People with GERD should also avoid eating large meals, and should instead eat several small meals throughout the day. It is also important to avoid lying down immediately after eating, as this can exacerbate symptoms. People with GERD can also help themselves by taking medication. Over-the-counter antacids can provide relief from mild symptoms. If symptoms are more severe, prescription medication may be necessary. People with GERD should also take care to maintain a healthy weight, as being overweight can exacerbate symptoms. Living with GERD does not have to be difficult. With a little bit of care and attention, people with GERD can live just as long and healthy of a life as people without GERD.

What are the 4 types of GERD?

Gastroesophageal reflux disease (GERD) is a condition in which the contents of the stomach reflux back up into the esophagus. The esophagus is the tube that carries food from the mouth to the stomach. GERD can cause heartburn, which is a sensation of pain or discomfort in the chest. GERD can also cause other symptoms, such as coughing, wheezing, and difficulty swallowing. There are four types of GERD: erosive GERD, in which stomach acid damages the lining of the esophagus; Barrett's esophagus, in which the lining of the esophagus is replaced by tissue that is similar to the lining of the intestine; stricture, in which the lining of the esophagus is narrowed; and ulcer, in which a ulcer forms in the lining of the esophagus. Erosive GERD is the most common type of GERD. It is characterized by a burning sensation in the chest, known as heartburn. Heartburn is caused by stomach acid coming in contact with the lining of the esophagus. Over time, stomach acid can damage the lining of the esophagus, leading to inflammation and ulceration. Barrett's esophagus is a condition in which the lining of the esophagus is replaced by tissue that is similar to the lining of the intestine. This condition is caused by chronic exposure to stomach acid. Barrett's esophagus increases the risk of esophageal cancer. Stricture is a condition in which the lining of the esophagus is narrowed. This narrowing can be caused by scar tissue, inflammation, or ulceration. Stricture can make it difficult to swallow. Ulcer is a condition in which an ulcer forms in the lining of the esophagus. Ulcers are usually caused by an infection, such as Helicobacter pylori, or by the use of non-steroidal anti-inflammatory drugs (NSAIDs). Ulcers can cause bleeding and perforation of the esophagus.

How sick can GERD make you feel?

GERD, or gastroesophageal reflux disease, can cause a range of uncomfortable and potentially dangerous symptoms. In some cases, GERD can be so severe that it leads to intense pain, nausea, and vomiting. In other cases, GERD can cause chest pain, difficulty swallowing, and even bleeding. GERD is caused by a backup of stomach acid into the esophagus. This backup can happen when the opening between the stomach and esophagus relaxes or widens, or when the stomach produces too much acid. GERD symptoms can range from mild to severe, and can vary from person to person. Some people with GERD may only experience a few episodes of heartburn, while others may have more frequent and more severe symptoms. The most common symptom of GERD is heartburn, which is a burning sensation in the chest. Other symptoms can include:

- Acid reflux - Chest pain - Difficulty swallowing - Nausea - Vomiting - Belching - Burping - Hiccups If you experience any of these symptoms, it's important to see a doctor. GERD can be a serious condition, and it's important to get treated as soon as possible.

How do you test for GERD?

There are a few ways to test for GERD. One way is an upper GI series, which is an x-ray of the esophagus, stomach, and intestines. Another way is endoscopy, which is a procedure where a small camera is inserted through the mouth and into the stomach. This allows the doctor to see any damage to the esophagus or stomach. Lastly, a pH test can be done, which measures the amount of acid in the stomach.

There are many possible causes of acid reflux, and it can be a serious condition. If you think you have acid reflux, you should see a doctor to get a diagnosis and treatment.

How long does GERD take to heal?

Acid reflux, or GERD, can be a painful and frustrating condition. But how long does it take to heal? The answer depends on a few factors, including the severity of your GERD and how you treat it. Some people find that their GERD symptoms go away on their own after a few weeks or months. Others may need medication or lifestyle changes to find relief. If your GERD is mild, you may be able to treat it with lifestyle changes, such as avoiding spicy foods, eating smaller meals, or not eating close to bedtime. If these changes don't help, your doctor may prescribe a medication to reduce stomach acid. If you have moderate or severe GERD, you may need to take a stronger medication to reduce stomach acid. You may also need to make lifestyle changes, such as losing weight, avoiding trigger foods, and not eating close to bedtime. Surgery may be an option for severe GERD that doesn't respond to other treatments. No matter what treatment you choose, it's important to keep working with your doctor to find the best way to relieve your symptoms. With the right treatment, you can find relief from your GERD and get back to enjoying your life.

What is the best GERD medicine?

There are a lot of different medicines that can be used to treat GERD, and it can be tough to decide which one is right for you. There are a few things that you can keep in mind when choosing a GERD medicine, and these tips will help you make the best decision for your needs. The first thing to consider is the severity of your GERD. If you have mild GERD, you might be able to get away with using an over-the-counter medication. However, if you have moderate or severe GERD, you'll likely need a prescription medication. Your doctor can help you decide which medication is right for you, and they will also take into consideration any other medications you're taking. That's because some GERD medicines can interact with other drugs, so it's important to be aware of that before you start taking anything. Another thing to keep in mind is that not all GERD medicines work the same way. Some medicines are designed to treat the symptoms of GERD, while others are designed to prevent it. So, if you're looking for a medicine that will keep you from having any GERD symptoms, you might need to try a few different medications before you find the one that works best for you. Finally, it's important to remember that GERD is a chronic condition, which means you'll likely need to take medication for it on a long-term basis. With that in mind, you'll want to choose a medication that is safe for long-term use and that you can afford. If you're not sure which GERD medicine is right for you, talk to your doctor. They can help you figure out the best option for your needs.

Does drinking water help GERD?

There are a lot of home remedies out there for dealing with gastrointestinal distress, and one of the most common is drinking water. But does water actually help with GERD? The simple answer is yes, but it depends on the circumstances. Drinking water can help to relieve symptoms of GERD for a couple of reasons. First of all, it can help to wash away any acid that has refluxed into the esophagus. This is because water is a natural neutralizer of acids. Secondly, water can also help to increase the production of saliva. This is important because saliva is one of the body's natural defenses against acid reflux. Saliva is alkaline, which means it can neutralize acids. So, the more saliva you have, the more protected you will be against the effects of GERD. Of course, there are other things you can do to help relieve symptoms of GERD, such as avoiding trigger foods, losing weight, and not smoking. But if you are looking for a simple and cheap home remedy, drinking water is a good place to start.

What is the difference between GERD and acid reflux?

GERD, or gastroesophageal reflux disease, and acid reflux are often used interchangeably, but there is a difference between the two. Acid reflux is a symptom of GERD, but GERD is a more serious, chronic condition. Acid reflux occurs when stomach acid rises up into the esophagus. This can happen after eating a large meal or drinking coffee or alcohol. Acid reflux is uncomfortable, and it can cause damage to the esophagus over time. GERD is a more serious condition that can lead to acid reflux. GERD occurs when the lower esophageal sphincter (LES) does not close properly, which allows stomach acid to leak back up into the esophagus. This can come and go, or it can be a chronic problem. GERD can cause damage to the esophagus, and it can also lead to other health problems. GERD can be treated with lifestyle changes, such as avoiding trigger foods and eating smaller meals. Medications can also be used to treat GERD, and in some cases, surgery may be necessary.

Is banana good for acid reflux?

There are a number of fruit choices that can help when you have acid reflux, and banana is one of them. Banana is known to be a good source of natural antacids, which can help to neutralize the acid in your stomach. Banana can also help to coat the lining of your stomach, which can help to protect it from the acid. When choosing a banana, make sure that it is ripe, as this will be the most effective. You can also eat banana with other food, such as oatmeal, which can also help to soothe your stomach. If you find that banana doesn't help, or you have other symptoms, such as heartburn, then you should speak to your doctor, as there may be other underlying causes.

Is Milk good for acid reflux?

It's no secret that milk can provide relief from heartburn and acid reflux. Milk is rich in calcium and also contains a small amount of sodium bicarbonate, which acts as an antacid to neutralize stomach acids. However, milk also contains lactic acid and casein, which can trigger or worsen symptoms in some people. So, is milk good or bad for acid reflux? It depends on the individual. Some people find that milk provides temporary relief from their symptoms, while others find that it makes their symptoms worse. If you're not sure whether milk is good or bad for you, it's best to try it and see how you feel. If you find that milk does help to relieve your symptoms, there are a few things you can do to make it even more effective. First, try drinking skim milk or low-fat milk instead of whole milk. Fat takes longer to digest and can make your symptoms worse. Also, try drinking milk with a meal instead of on an empty stomach. Milk can help to buffer the stomach acids and provide relief. But if you drink milk on an empty stomach, the acid can work its way up into the esophagus and trigger symptoms. If you find that milk doesn't help your symptoms or makes them worse, there are other things you can try. There are a number of non-dairy beverages that can provide relief, such as ginger ale, seltzer water, and decaffeinated coffee. You can also try taking an antacid.There are a variety of over-the-counter antacids available, such as Tums and Rolaids. If your symptoms are severe or don't improve with home treatment, it's important to see your doctor. You may have a more serious condition, such as GERD, and your doctor can recommend the best course of treatment.

Can GERD cause anxiety?

GERD, or gastroesophageal reflux disease, is a chronic and often severe condition in which stomach contents—including acid and sometimes bile—back up into the esophagus. This can cause symptoms like heartburn, chest pain, and shortness of breath. GERD can also lead to other, more serious health problems over time, such as esophageal cancer. While GERD on its own doesn't cause anxiety, the two conditions are often linked. Anxiety can make GERD symptoms worse, and GERD can trigger anxiety attacks. This can create a vicious cycle in which anxiety and GERD symptoms feed off of each other. There are a few possible explanations for why anxiety and GERD might be linked. First, chronic stress and anxiety can lead to changes in the nervous system that make you more sensitive to pain. This can make the symptoms of GERD, like heartburn and chest pain, feel more intense. Second, anxiety can affect the muscles in the digestive system, leading to changes that make it more likely for stomach contents to reflux into the esophagus. If you have both anxiety and GERD, it's important to seek treatment for both conditions. Treating one condition may help ease symptoms of the other. For example, if anxiety is making your GERD symptoms worse, treating your anxiety may help improve your GERD. Similarly, if GERD is triggering anxiety attacks, treating your GERD may help reduce your anxiety. There are a variety of treatments available for both anxiety and GERD. If you think you may have both conditions, talk to your doctor about the best treatment options for you.

Acid reflux is a condition in which stomach acid flows back up into the esophagus, causing heartburn and other symptoms. Treatments include lifestyle changes, medication, and surgery. While acid reflux can be uncomfortable, it is usually not a serious condition.

What foods heal GERD?

There are many food options that can heal GERD. Here are some examples of GERD-healing foods: 1. suspenseful fruits and vegetables such as bananas, melons, papayas, and root vegetables like carrots, sweet potatoes, and beets; 2. high-fiber foods such as whole grains, legumes, and Brussels sprouts; 3. low-fat proteins like skinless chicken, fish, and tofu; 4. probiotic-rich foods such as yogurt, sauerkraut, and kimchi; 5. herbal teas like ginger, fennel, and licorice root tea; 6. water, preferably alkaline water with a pH of 7.5 or higher. In addition to incorporating these GERD-healing foods into your diet, it is also important to avoid trigger foods that can exacerbate GERD symptoms. Common trigger foods include: 1. caffeinated beverages like coffee, tea, and soda; 2. alcohol; 3. fatty and fried foods; 4. spicy foods; 5. citrus fruits and juices; 6. tomatoes and tomato-based products; 7. mint; 8. garlic; 9. onions; 10. Chocolate. If you suffer from GERD, it is important to work with a healthcare professional to create a holistic treatment plan that includes both dietary and lifestyle changes. With the right changes, you can find relief from your GERD symptoms and heal your body.

What things make GERD worse?

There are a few things that make GERD, or gastroesophageal reflux disease, worse. One is eating too much. When you eat a lot, your stomach has to produce more acid to digest it all, and that can lead to heartburn. Another is eating certain foods. Some foods, like citrus fruits, tomatoes, chocolate, and caffeine, can make heartburn worse. Other things that can make GERD worse are being overweight, smoking, and drinking alcohol. Being overweight puts extra pressure on your stomach, which can cause acid to reflux. Smoking relaxes the valve between the stomach and esophagus, which can also lead to acid reflux. Drinking alcohol also relaxes the valve between the stomach and esophagus and can also increase the amount of acid your stomach produces. There are also some medical conditions that can make GERD worse. One is pregnancy. The extra weight from the baby can put pressure on the stomach and cause acid reflux. Another is a hiatal hernia. This is when the opening in the diaphragm that the esophagus goes through is too large. This can allow acid to come up from the stomach into the esophagus. GERD is a common condition, and there are things you can do to make it better. Avoiding triggering foods, maintaining a healthy weight, and not smoking are all good ways to help lessen the symptoms of GERD. If these things don't help, there are also medications that can be taken to help control the acid in your stomach.

What can I drink at night for acid reflux?

There are many things that people with acid reflux can do to help lessen their symptoms. One of those things is to avoid eating or drinking certain foods and drinks that trigger their acid reflux. For some people, that means avoiding acidic foods and drinks, such as citrus fruits, tomatoes, and coffee. For others, it might mean avoiding spicy foods, fatty foods, or anything else that seems to trigger their symptoms. There are also a few things that people with acid reflux can drink at night to help lessen their symptoms. One of those things is almond milk. Almond milk is a mildly alkaline drink that can help balance out the acidity in your stomach and lessen your symptoms. Another option is herbal tea. There are a number of different herbal teas that can be helpful for people with acid reflux, including ginger tea, chamomile tea, and licorice tea. If you're not sure what might trigger your acid reflux, or if you're looking for more ideas on how to lessen your symptoms, talk to your doctor or a registered dietitian.

What are red flags for GERD?

What are red flags for GERD? The most common symptom of gastroesophageal reflux disease (GERD) is chronic heartburn. Heartburn is a burning sensation in the chest that often occurs after eating. Other symptoms of GERD include: - regurgitation (a sour or bitter-tasting liquid coming back up into the throat or mouth) - difficulty swallowing - a dry cough - bad breath If you experience one or more of these symptoms regularly, it could be a sign of GERD. GERD can be a serious condition if left untreated. In some cases, it can lead to other medical problems such as ulcers, Barrett's esophagus (a precancerous condition), and even cancer of the esophagus. If you think you may have GERD, it's important to see your doctor for a diagnosis. They can recommend the best treatment for you. There are a few other conditions that can cause similar symptoms to GERD. These include esophageal spasm, gastritis, and peptic ulcers. Esophageal spasm is a condition that causes the muscles in the esophagus to contract abnormally. This can lead to symptoms such as chest pain, difficulty swallowing, and regurgitation. Gastritis is an inflammation of the stomach lining. It can cause symptoms such as stomach pain, nausea, and vomiting. Peptic ulcers are sores that develop on the lining of the stomach or duodenum (the first part of the small intestine). They can cause symptoms such as abdominal pain, heartburn, and nausea. If you experience any of the above symptoms, it's important to see your doctor to rule out any serious conditions.

What happens if you have GERD for too long?

GERD, or gastroesophageal reflux disease, is a condition in which the contents of the stomach — namely, acid and digestive juices — back up into the esophagus. This can cause a burning sensation in the chest or throat, commonly known as heartburn. Most people experience occasional heartburn, and it is generally not a cause for concern. However, when heartburn occurs more than twice a week, it may be a sign of GERD. If GERD is left untreated, it can lead to serious complications, such as: - Esophageal stricture: This is a narrowing of the esophagus caused by damage from the acid reflux. - Barrett's esophagus: This is a condition in which the lining of the esophagus is replaced by tissue that is similar to the lining of the intestine. This is a precancerous condition. - Esophageal adenocarcinoma: This is a rare but serious type of cancer that occurs in the esophageal lining. If you think you may have GERD, it is important to see your doctor. They can offer lifestyle changes that may help to lessen your symptoms, such as avoiding trigger foods and eating smaller meals. In some cases, medication may be necessary to control the symptoms of GERD.

How do I know if my esophagus is damaged?

The term "acid reflux" refers to the backward flow of stomach contents, including acids, into the esophagus. This can happen when the lower esophageal sphincter (LES), a muscle that acts as a valve between the esophagus and stomach, does not close properly. Acid reflux can cause heartburn, a painful sensation in the chest. Heartburn occurs when stomach acids back up into the esophagus, the tube that carries food from the mouth to the stomach. Certain foods, such as fried or fatty foods, citrus fruits, chocolate, caffeine, and carbonated beverages, can make heartburn worse. Heartburn is not the only symptom of acid reflux. Other symptoms include: -Chest pain -Difficulty swallowing -Dry cough -Hoarseness -Sore throat -Regurgitation of food or sour liquid -Bad breath If you experience any of these symptoms, it is important to see your doctor, as they may be indicative of a more serious condition, such as gastroesophageal reflux disease (GERD) or a hiatal hernia. GERD is a chronic form of acid reflux that can damage the esophagus and lead to other complications, such as Barrett's esophagus. A hiatal hernia occurs when part of the stomach protrudes through the diaphragm, the muscle that separates the chest and abdominal cavities. Esophageal damage from acid reflux can lead to bleeding, ulcers, and scarring. These can result in difficulty swallowing or, in severe cases, choking. If you experience any of the following symptoms, you should seek medical attention immediately, as they may indicate a more serious condition: -Vomiting blood -Black stools -Difficulty breathing -Chest pain that spreads to the jaw, neck, or arm -Sudden onset of hoarseness If you think you may have acid reflux, it is important to see your doctor, as the condition can be treated. Left untreated, however, acid reflux can lead to serious complications.

What causes gastroesophageal reflux disease?

Acid reflux disease, also known as GERD, is a condition in which the contents of the stomach escape backwards into the esophagus. The stomach contents are very acidic, and this can cause damage to the esophagus. There are a number of things that can contribute to acid reflux disease. One is diet. Certain foods can trigger the production of acid in the stomach, and if you eat a lot of these foods, you may be more likely to experience acid reflux. Some of the most common trigger foods include coffee, chocolate, fatty foods, and citrus fruits. Another factor that can contribute to acid reflux disease is a hiatal hernia. This is a condition in which part of the stomach protrudes through the diaphragm into the chest cavity. This can cause the contents of the stomach to press against the esophageal sphincter, making it more likely for acid to escape into the esophagus. There are also a number of medical conditions that can increase your risk for acid reflux disease. These include pregnancy, diabetes, and certain types of infections. If you think you may be suffering from acid reflux disease, it's important to see your doctor. They can diagnose the condition and recommend the best course of treatment.

Acid reflux is a condition that can be caused by a number of things, including diet, lifestyle, and medications. If you suffer from acid reflux, you may want to consider making some changes to your diet and lifestyle. There are also a number of medications that can help to control or eliminate acid reflux.

What are the warning signs of GERD?

There are a few all-too-common symptoms associated with GERD: heartburn, chest pain, and trouble swallowing. But did you know that GERD can also cause other less-recognized symptoms? Here are some potential warning signs that you may have GERD: 1. A sour taste in your mouth. This is caused by stomach acid backing up into your esophagus. 2.Bad breath. This is also caused by stomach acid backing up into your esophagus. 3. A hoarse voice. This is caused by stomach acid irritating your vocal cords. 4. A chronic cough. This is caused by stomach acid irritating your airways. 5. Wheezing. This is also caused by stomach acid irritating your airways. 6. Chest pain. This is caused by stomach acid irritating your esophagus. 7. Trouble swallowing. This is caused by stomach acid damaging your esophagus. 8. A feeling of food stuck in your throat. This is also caused by stomach acid damaging your esophagus. 9. Nausea. This is caused by stomach acid irritating your stomach. 10. Vomiting. This is also caused by stomach acid irritating your stomach. If you experience any of these symptoms, it's important to see your doctor. GERD is a serious condition that can lead to long-term damage to your esophagus if left untreated.

How do you fix gastroesophageal reflux disease?

The most common treatment for gastroesophageal reflux disease (GERD) is a type of medication called a proton pump inhibitor (PPI). PPIs work by blocking the production of stomach acid. This can help to relieve the symptoms of GERD, such as heartburn, chest pain, and difficulty swallowing. There are a variety of PPIs available, and they are often used in combination with other medications, such as antacids. PPIs are generally considered to be safe, but there are some potential side effects, such as headache, diarrhea, and nausea. If PPIs are not effective in treating GERD, other medications, such as H2 blockers or prokinetics, may be recommended. Surgery is also an option for severe cases of GERD that do not respond to medical treatment.

What happens if GERD is left untreated?

GERD, or gastroesophageal reflux disease, is a chronic condition characterized by frequent episodes of acid reflux. If left untreated, GERD can lead to serious complications, such as esophageal ulcers, esophageal strictures, and even esophageal cancer. The most common symptom of GERD is heartburn, which is a burning sensation in the chest that can extend to the throat. Other symptoms include regurgitation, dysphagia, and chest pain. GERD is caused by a malfunctioning of the lower esophageal sphincter (LES), a ring of muscle that separates the esophagus from the stomach. Normally, the LES relaxes to allow food and liquids to pass into the stomach, and then contracts to prevent backflow into the esophagus. In people with GERD, the LES either relaxes too much or does not contract properly, allowing stomach contents to flow back into the esophagus. There are several factors that can contribute to the development of GERD, including obesity, pregnancy, smoking, and certain medications. Some medical conditions, such as hiatal hernia, can also cause or worsen GERD. Treatment for GERD typically involves lifestyle changes, such as eating smaller meals and avoiding trigger foods. Medications, such as antacids, proton pump inhibitors, and H2 blockers, can also be used to reduce the symptoms of GERD. In some cases, surgery may be necessary to repair the damage caused by GERD. If left untreated, GERD can lead to serious and even life-threatening complications. Esophageal ulcers are open sores that develop in the lining of the esophagus as a result of exposure to stomach acid. Ulcers can bleed, and may eventually lead to esophageal strictures, or narrowing of the esophagus. Esophageal cancer is another potential complication of GERD. While cancer of the esophagus is relatively rare, it is one of the most aggressive and deadly forms of cancer. GERD is a serious condition that can have potentially life-threatening consequences. If you experience any of the symptoms of GERD, it is important to see a doctor so that the condition can be properly diagnosed and treated.

What foods should you avoid with GERD?

If you suffer from gastroesophageal reflux disease (GERD), you may find your symptoms aggravated by what you eat. There are certain foods that can trigger GERD symptoms and it is important to be aware of which foods these are so that you can avoid them. Certain foods are known to trigger GERD symptoms by causing the lower esophageal sphincter to relax or by increasing the amount of acid in the stomach. Foods that commonly trigger GERD symptoms include: -Citrus fruits such as oranges, lemons and grapefruit -Tomatoes and tomato-based products -Spicy foods

-Fatty and fried foods -Coffee and tea -Chocolate -Alcohol You may find that you are sensitive to one or more of these foods and that avoiding them helps to reduce your GERD symptoms. Keep a food diary to help identify which foods trigger your symptoms so that you can avoid them. In addition to avoiding trigger foods, there are a few other dietary changes that can help to reduce GERD symptoms. Eating smaller, more frequent meals instead of large meals can help to reduce the amount of acid in the stomach. Avoiding eating close to bedtime can also help, as lying down after eating can allow acid to reflux from the stomach into the esophagus. finally, losing weight if you are overweight can also help to reduce GERD symptoms.

Will GERD go away?

Gastroesophageal reflux disease, or GERD, is a condition where the contents of the stomach come back up into the esophagus. This can cause heartburn, chest pain, and other symptoms. GERD is a chronic condition, which means it can last a long time. Some people only have mild symptoms, while others may have more severe symptoms. There is no cure for GERD, but there are treatments that can help lessen the symptoms. In some cases, GERD may go away on its own.

How long does Gastroesophageal reflux last?

Gastroesophageal reflux, also known as GERD or acid reflux, is a common condition in which stomach contents rise up into the esophagus. Symptoms include heartburn, chest pain, and regurgitation. GERD is usually diagnosed based on symptoms and sometimes a diagnostic test called an upper GI series. Most people with GERD will experience symptoms for a few months to a few years and then the symptoms will go away. In some people, however, GERD can be a chronic, lifelong condition. There is no cure for GERD, but treatments are available to help control the symptoms. The most common symptom of GERD is heartburn. Heartburn is a burning sensation in the chest that can be caused by stomach acid rising up into the esophagus. Other symptoms of GERD include: –Chest pain –Regurgitation –Difficulty swallowing –Hoarseness –Coughing –Sore throat If you experience any of these symptoms, it is important to see your doctor to rule out other possible causes. GERD is usually diagnosed based on symptoms and sometimes a diagnostic test called an upper GI series. There is no cure for GERD, but treatments are available to help control the symptoms. The goal of treatment is to reduce the symptoms and prevent complications. Lifestyle changes are often the first line of treatment for GERD. These changes can include: –Eating smaller meals –Eliminating foods that trigger symptoms –Avoiding eating late at night –avoiding tight-fitting clothing –maintaining a healthy weight –quitting smoking – avoiding lying down for three hours after eating If lifestyle changes do not improve the symptoms of GERD, your doctor may recommend medications. The most common medications used to treat GERD are: –Antacids: Antacids neutralize stomach acid and can provide quick relief. –H2 blockers: H2 blockers reduce the production of stomach acid. –Proton pump inhibitors: Proton pump inhibitors are the most effective type of medication for GERD. They work by reducing the production of stomach acid. Surgery is an option for people who do not respond to lifestyle changes or medications. Surgery is usually only recommended for people with severe GERD who are at risk for complications. If you have GERD, it is important to see your doctor to discuss your treatment options. With treatment, most people with GERD can control their symptoms and live normal, healthy lives.

When should I see a doctor for GERD?

Certain symptoms may signal that your acid reflux is more serious and requires medical attention. If you experience any of the following, it's time to see a doctor: Frequent, severe heartburn An inability to swallow Weight loss Vomiting Black stools GERD is a chronic condition, and its symptoms can be controlled in most cases. However, some people may develop complications, such as esophageal ulcers or Barrett's esophagus. These conditions can increase your risk of esophageal cancer. If you have any concerns about your acid reflux, make an appointment to see your doctor.

In conclusion, acid reflux is a condition that can be effectively managed with lifestyle changes and medication. With a little bit of effort, you can control your acid reflux and enjoy your life free from the uncomfortable symptoms.

How do you know if your acid is high?

Acid reflux can be difficult to diagnose because it presents similarly to other digestive disorders and its symptoms can be vague. However, there are certain tell-tale signs that can help you determine if your acid reflux is indeed high. These include: Heartburn: This is the most classic symptom of acid reflux and is characterized by a burning sensation in the chest, often after eating. Acid regurgitation: This is when stomach acid actually comes up into the mouth and can leave a sour, bitter taste. Dyspepsia: This is a general term for discomfort or pain in the stomach area. It can be accompanied by bloating, belching, and nausea. GI problems: Acid reflux is often linked with other GI disorders such as ulcers and Crohn's disease. If you have any of these conditions, it's likely that your acid reflux is high. If you experience any of these symptoms on a regular basis, it's important to see a doctor so that they can properly diagnose and treat your acid reflux. Left untreated, acid reflux can lead to serious complications such as esophageal damage or even cancer. So, don't hesitate to seek help if you think your acid reflux may be high.

Can Gaviscon help with GERD?

Acid reflux is a condition in which stomach acid rises up into the esophagus, causing heartburn and other uncomfortable symptoms. Gaviscon is a medication that is used to treat heartburn and other symptoms of acid reflux. Gaviscon works by forming a barrier between the stomach and the esophagus. This barrier prevents stomach acid from coming up into the esophagus and causing heartburn and other uncomfortable symptoms. There is some evidence that Gaviscon can help to reduce the symptoms of GERD. However, it is important to remember that Gaviscon is not a cure for GERD and it is important to talk to your doctor about the best way to treat your condition.

Are bananas OK for GERD?

Are bananas good for GERD? This is a common question asked by those who suffer from the condition. While there is no clear-cut answer, some say that bananas may help ease symptoms while others find them to make GERD worse. Let's take a closer look at the pros and cons of eating bananas for GERD. On the plus side, bananas are a low-acid fruit, which means they won't trigger your symptoms as much as other foods. They're also a good source of fiber, which can help keep you regular and improve your digestion. And, since bananas are mild and easily digestible, they may be a good choice if you're feeling especially sensitive. On the downside, some people find that bananas aggravate their symptoms. This may be because they're a high-carbohydrate food, which can lead to gas and bloating. Bananas are also relatively high in sugar, which can promote the growth of bacteria in your gut. If you're looking to limit your sugar intake, you may want to avoid bananas or eat them in moderation. So, what's the verdict? If you have GERD, you'll need to experiment to see what works for you. Start by trying a small piece of banana and see how you feel. If it doesn't bother you, you can gradually add more to your diet. Just be sure to listen to your body and stop eating if you start to feel any discomfort.

What are the best snacks for acid reflux?

There are a few things to consider when choosing snacks if you suffer from acid reflux. You want to avoid anything that is going to trigger your reflux, so stay away from fatty or fried foods, as well as anything spicy, citrusy, or with caffeine. You also want to avoid lying down directly after eating, so choose snacks that are easy to digest. With that in mind, here are a few ideas for snacks that should be easy on your stomach and won't trigger your acid reflux: Plain popcorn is a great option for a light, easy-to-digest snack. Just be sure to avoid the buttery, salty kind you get at the movies. Plain yogurt or kefir is another good choice. Look for brands that are low in fat and sugar, and top with fresh fruit or a small amount of honey for sweetness. A handful of nuts is a filling snack that's easy on the stomach. Just be sure to avoid ones that are high in acid, like walnuts or cashews. A slice of whole-wheat bread with a bit of peanut butter is another satisfying option. If you're looking for something sweet, a small piece of dark chocolate is a good choice. Just be sure to avoid chocolate that is high in milk or sugar, as these can trigger reflux. These are just a few ideas for snacks that won't trigger your acid reflux. Of course, you should talk to your doctor about what foods are best for you to eat.

Can I drink coffee with GERD?

GERD, or gastroesophageal reflux disease, is a condition that causes stomach acid to rise up into the esophagus. This can cause a burning sensation in the chest or throat, and can even lead to damage of the esophagus if it is not treated. Many people with GERD find that their symptoms are worse after eating, and so they may wonder if it is safe to drink coffee with GERD. Coffee is acidic, and so it can aggravate symptoms of GERD. However, everyone's body is different, and so coffee may not have the same effect on everyone with GERD. Some people find that their symptoms are worsened by coffee, while others find that it does not make a difference. If you are not sure whether coffee affects your GERD, you may want to try avoiding it for a week or two to see if your symptoms improve. There are also a few things you can do to make coffee less likely to trigger GERD symptoms. Adding milk or cream to your coffee can help to neutralize the acidity, and drinking decaffeinated coffee may also be less likely to trigger symptoms. If you find that coffee does aggravate your GERD, you may want to limit your intake or switch to herbal tea instead.

Is GERD a symptom of anxiety?

GERD, or gastroesophageal reflux disease, is a common condition in which stomach contents rise up into the esophagus. This can cause symptoms such as heartburn, chest pain, and a sour taste in the mouth. Many people with GERD also have anxiety, and the two conditions may be linked. Anxiety is a common mood disorder that can cause a variety of symptoms, including feelings of worry, fear, and unease. People with anxiety may also experience physical symptoms such as a racing heart, sweating, and difficulty breathing. When someone has both GERD and anxiety, the symptoms can be magnified. GERD and anxiety may be linked in several ways. Anxiety can lead to behaviors that can aggravate GERD, such as overeating, eating spicy or fatty foods, and drinking alcohol. Anxiety can also cause changes in the way the digestive system works, which can lead to inflammation and changes in the sensitivity of the esophagus. Treatment for GERD and anxiety often includes lifestyle changes, such as taking steps to reduce stress, eating a balanced diet, and avoiding trigger foods. In some cases, medication may also be necessary. If you have GERD and anxiety, talk to your doctor about the best way to manage both conditions.

Can lack of sleep cause acid reflux?

It is well known that a good night's sleep is crucial for our overall health and well-being. But what many people don't realize is that sleep can also have a significant impact on our digestive system and, specifically, can either help to relieve or cause acid reflux. There are a few ways in which sleep can affect acid reflux. First, when we are lying down, gravity is no longer working in our favor to keep food and stomach acid where they belong – in our stomachs. Instead, everything is much more likely to come back up towards the esophagus. Second, when we are asleep, we are more likely to swallow less often, which gives stomach acid more opportunities to travel back up the esophagus. And finally, sleep is a time when our body's overall relaxed state can lead to a relaxation of the lower esophageal sphincter, the muscle that keeps stomach acid where it belongs. So, if you suffer from acid reflux, it is important to make sure that you are getting enough sleep. aim for at least 7-8 hours per night. In addition, there are a few other things you can do to help reduce the likelihood of acid reflux at night: -Avoid eating large meals close to bedtime -Don't lie down immediately after eating -Elevate your head and torso when you sleep

Acid reflux is a condition in which the stomach contents are regurgitated up into the esophagus. This can happen when the lower esophageal sphincter, which is a muscle that separates the stomach from the esophagus, does not close properly. Acid reflux can be painful and may cause problems such as heartburn, chest pain, and trouble swallowing. There are many treatments available to help relieve the symptoms of acid reflux.

Can silent reflux cause panic attacks?

While there is no one definitive answer to this question, it is possible that silent reflux may play a role in panic attacks for some people. For example, if someone experiences silent reflux regularly, the constant contact of stomach acid with the throat and esophagus may eventually lead to inflammation. This inflammation can cause a variety of symptoms, including anxiety and panic. Additionally, the pain and discomfort associated with silent reflux may also trigger a panic attack. It is important to note that silent reflux is just one potential cause of panic attacks. There are many other possible causes, including genetics, stress, and other medical conditions. If you are experience panic attacks, it is important to talk to a doctor or mental health professional to determine the cause and develop a treatment plan.

Is yogurt good for acid reflux?

Acid reflux is a condition in which stomach acids back up into the esophagus, causing a burning sensation in the chest or throat. Some people believe that yogurt may help to relieve symptoms of acid reflux, but there is no scientific evidence to support this claim. Yogurt is a fermented dairy product that contains live and active cultures, or probiotics. Probiotics are beneficial bacteria that can improve gut health. Some research suggests that probiotics may help to reduce the symptoms of acid reflux. A small study in 2017 found that yogurt improved reflux symptoms in people with laryngopharyngeal reflux, a type of acid reflux that affects the throat. However, more research is needed to determine whether yogurt is effective for treating other types of acid reflux. There is no evidence to suggest that yogurt is an effective treatment for acid reflux. However, some research indicates that probiotics, which are found in yogurt, may help to relieve symptoms. If you're considering adding yogurt to your diet, talk to your doctor first to see if it's right for you.

What is the best probiotic for silent reflux?

The best probiotic for silent reflux is one that is high in quality and has been proven to be effective. There are a few different brands that make these types of probiotics, and they can be found in both pill and powder form. The most important thing is to find one that is right for you and that you feel comfortable taking. If you are someone who suffers from silent reflux, you know how frustrating and embarrassing it can be. You might be wondering what you can do to get rid of it. There are a few different ways to treat silent reflux. One way is to take a probiotic. Probiotics are live bacteria that are good for your gut. They can help to restore the balance of bacteria in your gut, which can help to reduce the symptoms of silent reflux. Probiotics can be found in both pill and powder form. Another way to treat silent reflux is to make some changes to your diet. Avoiding trigger foods is a good place to start. Common trigger foods include fatty foods, spicy foods, chocolate, caffeine, and alcohol. If you are not sure what your trigger foods are, you can keep a food diary to help you identify them. You should also avoid eating late at night and lying down after eating. There are a few other things you can do to help reduce the symptoms of silent reflux. One is to prop up your head when you sleep. This can help to reduce the amount of acid that refluxes into your esophagus. You can also try to avoid tight-fitting clothing. This can help to reduce the pressure on your stomach and make it less likely that acid will reflux. If you smoke, quitting is also a good idea. Smoking can irritate your esophagus and make symptoms worse. If you have tried all of these things and you are still having symptoms, you may want to talk to your doctor about medication. There are a few different types of medication that can be used to treat silent reflux. One type is called PPIs. These work by reducing the amount of acid that your stomach produces. Another type of medication is H2 blockers. These work by blocking the histamine receptor, which can help to reduce the amount of acid that is produced. If you are dealing with silent reflux, know that you are not alone. This is a very common condition. But, there are things that you can do to help reduce the symptoms. Talk to your doctor about what might be the best option for you.

Is Yakult drink good for acid reflux?

Is Yakult drink good for acid reflux? Acid reflux is a condition in which the contents of the stomach regurgitate up into the esophagus, causing heartburn and other painful symptoms. There are many potential causes of acid reflux, such as overeating, eating spicy or fatty foods, and lying down after eating. Yakult is a Probiotic drink that is widely promoted as being helpful for digestive health. The drink contains live bacteria that are thought to aid in the digestion of food. Some people believe that Yakult can also help to reduce the symptoms of acid reflux. There is some evidence to support the use of Yakult for acid reflux. A study published in the Journal of Gastroenterology and Hepatology found that people who drank Yakult had a lower risk of developing acid reflux symptoms. However, it is important to remember that Yakult is not a cure for acid reflux. If you are experiencing symptoms of acid reflux, it is important to see a doctor to find out the cause and to receive treatment. While Yakult may be helpful for some people with acid reflux, it is not a guaranteed cure. If you are concerned about your acid reflux symptoms, it is important to speak with a doctor to find out the cause and to receive the best treatment for your individual case.

What vitamin deficiencies cause acid reflux?

Acid reflux, commonly referred to as GERD, or gastroesophageal reflux disease, is a condition in which the contents of the stomach are returned to the esophagus, causing a burning sensation in the chest or throat. While acid reflux can be aggravated by certain foods and lifestyle choices, it can also be a symptom of a vitamin deficiency. Here are some of the most common vitamin deficiencies that can cause acid reflux: Vitamin B12: Also known as cobalamin, vitamin B12 is essential for the proper function of the nervous system and for the production of red blood cells. A vitamin B12 deficiency can lead to anemia, which is a common cause of acid reflux. Vitamin D: Vitamin D is essential for calcium absorption and for maintaining bone health. A vitamin D deficiency can lead to osteoporosis, which can contribute to acid reflux by weakening the esophageal sphincter. Vitamin C: Vitamin C is an important antioxidant that helps to protect the body from damage caused by free radicals. A vitamin C deficiency can weaken the immune system, making the body more susceptible to infections, which can lead to acid reflux. While these are the most common vitamin deficiencies that can cause acid reflux, there are other less common deficiencies that can also contribute to the condition. These include deficiencies in iron, magnesium, and zinc. If you think you may be suffering from a vitamin deficiency, talk to your doctor about being tested and starting a supplement regimen.

Does Gaviscon Advance work for LPR?

Gaviscon Advance is a medication that is used to treat heartburn and acid reflux. It is a over-the-counter medication that is available in liquid and tablet form. The active ingredient in Gaviscon Advance is aluminum hydroxide, which works to neutralize stomach acid. There is limited research on the effectiveness of Gaviscon Advance for treating GERD or LPR. One study found that Gaviscon Advance was not effective in reducing the symptoms of GERD in a group of children. However, another study found that Gaviscon Advance was effective in treating LPR in a group of adults. If you are considering using Gaviscon Advance for the treatment of GERD or LPR, you should speak with your doctor first. Gaviscon Advance is generally considered safe, but there are some potential side effects, such as constipation, diarrhea, and bleeding.

Acid reflux affects millions of Americans every year. While there are many over-the-counter and prescription treatments available, many people opt for natural remedies. Changing your diet, avoiding trigger foods, and managing stress can help control acid reflux and keep symptoms to a minimum.

Why am I getting reflux all of a sudden?

There are many possible explanations for why you might suddenly start experiencing acid reflux. One possibility is that you have developed a food intolerance or are eating foods that trigger reflux. Another possibility is that you have a medical condition such as gastroesophageal reflux disease (GERD) or a hiatal hernia. Stress, smoking, and certain medications can also contribute to acid reflux. If you are concerned about why you are suddenly getting reflux, you should talk to your doctor to rule out any underlying medical causes.

How do I know what stage of GERD I have?

Acid reflux is a condition in which stomach acid flows back up into the esophagus, causing a burning sensation in the chest or throat. There are four stages of GERD, and each stage is characterized by different symptoms. Stage 1: This is the mildest stage of GERD. Symptoms include heartburn, which is a burning sensation in the chest or throat. Stage 2: This stage is characterized by more frequent and more severe symptoms. In addition to heartburn, symptoms may include regurgitation, which is when stomach acid and food flow back up into the throat. Stage 3: This is the most severe stage of GERD. In addition to heartburn and regurgitation, symptoms may include chest pain, difficulty swallowing, and even bleeding. Stage 4: This is the most severe and potentially life-threatening stage of GERD. In addition to the symptoms of the previous stages, symptoms may include severe chest pain, a fast heart rate, and difficulty breathing. If you experience any of these symptoms, you should seek medical attention immediately.

Can you be hospitalized for GERD?

Acid reflux, also known as GERD, is a common condition in which the stomach contents – including the acid – back up into the esophagus. This can cause a burning sensation in the chest or throat, as well as other symptoms. In some cases, acid reflux can lead to further complications, such as an erosion of the esophagus or even hospitalization.

How can I test my stomach acid at home?

There are a couple of ways that you can test your stomach acid at home. The first is to try a simple acidity test. You can do this by mixing together one cup of water and two tablespoons of apple cider vinegar. Then, drink the mixture on an empty stomach first thing in the morning. If you experience any burning or discomfort, that is a sign that you have low stomach acid levels. Another way to test your stomach acid is to take a supplement that contains hydrochloric acid. You can take this supplement before a meal, and if you experience any heartburn or indigestion, that is a sign that your stomach acid levels are low. If you want to be sure, you can talk to your doctor about having a test done to measure your stomach acid levels.

How long does it take for stomach acid to return to normal?

It usually takes about one to two hours for stomach acid levels to return to normal after eating. However, this may vary depending on the amount of food consumed and individual difference. Some factors that can contribute to how quickly stomach acidity returns to normal include the type of food consumed (fatty foods tend to slow down digestion), how well the food was chewed (food that is not well-chewed takes longer to digest), and how much water was consumed with the meal (water helps to dilute stomach acids).

What foods heal the esophagus?

There are certain foods that have been shown to help heal the esophagus and reduce the symptoms of acid reflux. These include: -Herbal tea: Herbal teas can help to soothe the digestive system and reduce inflammation. -Probiotic foods: Probiotic foods contain live bacteria that can help to balance the gut flora and reduce intestinal inflammation. -Fruits and vegetables: Fruits and vegetables are high in fiber and water content, both of which can help to bulk up the stool and reduce constipation. -Lean protein: Lean protein is easy to digest and can help to repair the lining of the gastrointestinal tract. -Olive oil: Olive oil contains healthy fats that can help to reduce inflammation throughout the body. If you suffer from acid reflux, it is important to talk to your doctor about which foods may be the best for you.

How can I repair my esophagus naturally?

There are a few things that you can do in order to repair your esophagus naturally. The first thing is to make sure that you are eating healthy and not overeating. When you overeat, it puts a lot of pressure on your stomach, which can cause your esophageal sphincter to relax and allow acid to come back up. Another thing to do is to avoid foods that are high in acid, such as citrus fruits, tomatoes, and spicy foods. You should also avoid drinking alcohol and smoking, as both of these can irritate your esophagus. Finally, make sure to get plenty of rest and exercise, as both of these can help to reduce stress and promote healing.

While over-the-counter and prescription medications are available to treat acid reflux, making lifestyle changes may be the best way to prevent it. Avoiding trigger foods, eating smaller meals, and avoiding eating late at night can help reduce the occurrence of acid reflux. Drinking plenty of water and staying upright after eating can also help.

How do I know if I have an ulcer in my esophagus?

If you think you might have an ulcer, it's important to see a doctor right away. An ulcer is a sore that forms in the lining of your stomach or the first part of your small intestine, called the duodenum. Ulcers develop when the acids that digest food wear away the protective lining of your stomach or duodenum. This can happen if: You have an infection with the Helicobacter pylori (H. pylori) bacteria. H. pylori is found in the stomach of about half of the world's population. In most cases, it does not cause any problems. But it is responsible for the majority of ulcers. You take pain relievers called nonsteroidal anti-inflammatory drugs (NSAIDs) on a regular basis. These include ibuprofen (Advil, Motrin) and naproxen (Aleve). You drink too much alcohol. You smoke. You have stress. While stress does not cause ulcers, it can make them worse. Most ulcers are not painful. But some people with ulcers experience a burning sensation in their stomach between meals. This feeling often occurs when the stomach is empty. It may be relieved by eating or taking antacids. Other people with ulcers have pain that feels like hunger. This pain may occur at any time and may get worse when your stomach is empty. It may be relieved by eating or taking antacids. Ulcers can also cause other symptoms, such as: Nausea Vomiting Loss of appetite Weight loss Bloating Burping If you have any of these symptoms, it's important to see a doctor. Only a doctor can tell for sure if you have an ulcer.

What are the 10 most acidic foods?

There are a variety of acidic foods that can trigger acid reflux, and it's important to know which ones to avoid. Here are 10 of the most acidic foods: 1. Citrus fruits: Oranges, lemons, and grapefruits are all high in acidity and can trigger acid reflux. 2. Tomatoes: While tomatoes are a healthy food, they are also highly acidic. 3. Coffee: Many people enjoy coffee first thing in the morning, but the acidity can trigger acid reflux. 4. Tea: Like coffee, tea can be acidic and trigger acid reflux. 5. Soda: Soda is often filled with empty calories and can be a trigger for acid reflux. 6. Alcohol: Alcohol can relax the esophageal sphincter, which can lead to acid reflux. 7. Spicy foods: Spicy foods can trigger acid reflux in some people. 8. Fatty foods: Fatty foods can slow down the digestion process and trigger acid reflux. 9. Processed foods: Processed foods are often high in fat and preservatives, both of which can trigger acid reflux. 10. Chocolate: Chocolate contains caffeine and theobromine, both of which can trigger acid reflux.

What foods absorb stomach acid?

If you have acid reflux, you know that certain foods can make your symptoms worse. If you're looking for foods that absorb stomach acid, you might be wondering which ones are the best choices. There are a few different ways that food can help to absorb stomach acid. One is by neutralizing the acid. This can be done by eating foods that are high in alkalinity, such as fruits and vegetables. Another way is by binding to the acid, which can help to reduce its effects. Foods that are high in fiber, such as whole grains, can help to do this. Fatty foods can also help to absorb stomach acid. This is because they slow down the emptying of the stomach, which gives the acid more time to be neutralized. However, fatty foods can also make acid reflux worse, so it's important to find a balance that works for you. In general, the best foods for acid reflux are those that are low in acidity and high in alkalinity. Fruits and vegetables are good choices, as are whole grains and fatty foods. Everyone is different, though, so it's important to experiment to see what works for you.

What foods help with acid reflux at night?

There are a few things you can do to ease acid reflux at night. First, avoid foods that trigger your reflux. Common triggers include spicy foods, fatty foods, citrus fruits, and tomatoes. If you're unsure what your triggers are, keep a food diary and note when your reflux flares up. You may also want to avoid eating late at night, as lying down after a meal can aggravate reflux. Instead, focus on foods that soothe your stomach and help neutralize acid. Good options include low-fat yogurt, bananas, oatmeal, and ginger. You can also try chewing on a piece of gum after meals to help keep acid at bay. If you still find yourself struggling with acid reflux at night, talk to your doctor about other potential treatments, such as lifestyle changes, medications, or surgery.

What drinks should I avoid with acid reflux?

There are a few drinks that you should avoid if you have acid reflux. These include carbonated beverages, alcohol, caffeinated drinks, and citrus juices. Drinking carbonated beverages can cause acid reflux because they increase the amount of acid in your stomach. This can lead to heartburn and other symptoms. Alcohol can also relax the lower esophageal sphincter, which can cause acid reflux. Caffeinated drinks, such as coffee and tea, can also trigger acid reflux. Citrus juices, such as orange and grapefruit juice, can also increase the amount of acid in your stomach.

Does honey and hot water help acid reflux?

When it comes to finding relief from the painful and uncomfortable symptoms of acid reflux, people are often willing to try anything. So, it's no surprise that one home remedy for acid reflux is honey and hot water. But does it really work? The short answer is that there is no definitive answer. Some people swear by the effectiveness of honey and hot water for acid reflux, while others find it does nothing to help. There is some evidence to suggest that honey may help to reduce the symptoms of acid reflux. One study found that honey was effective in reducing the amount of acid in the stomach and also in healing gastric ulcers. Another study found that a combination of honey and vinegar was effective in treating acid reflux. However, it's important to note that this study was conducted on rats, not humans. There is also some evidence to suggest that honey may have anti-inflammatory properties. This means it could potentially help to reduce the inflammation that is often associated with acid reflux. So, what does all this evidence mean? Well, it suggests that honey may help to reduce the symptoms of acid reflux in some people. However, it's important to remember that there is no definitive proof that honey is effective for treating acid reflux. If you're considering using honey to treat your acid reflux, it's important to speak to your doctor first. This is especially important if you're taking any medication for your acid reflux, as honey could potentially interact with your medication. Your doctor will be able to advise you on whether honey is a good option for you and, if so, how much you should take.

Does ice cream help acid reflux?

Acid reflux is a condition in which the stomach acid flows back up into the esophagus, causing a burning sensation in the chest or throat. Many people wonder if ice cream can help to relieve the symptoms of acid reflux. It is possible that ice cream may help to relieve the symptoms of acid reflux in some people. The cool temperature of the ice cream can help to soothe the burning sensation in the throat. The fat content in ice cream can also help to coat the lining of the esophagus, which may help to protect it from the stomach acid. However, it is important to remember that ice cream is also high in sugar and calories, which can contribute to weight gain. This can make acid reflux worse. So, if you are looking for a way to treat your acid reflux, you may want to try a low-fat or sugar-free option.

In conclusion, acid reflux can be a very uncomfortable and even dangerous condition if not treated properly. If you think you may be suffering from acid reflux, be sure to talk to your doctor to get a proper diagnosis and treatment plan.

Do sweets help with acid reflux?

Acid reflux can be a frustrating and painful condition, made worse by the fact that many of the foods we enjoy most are often the ones that trigger reflux symptoms. So it's no wonder that people with acid reflux often ask the question: do sweets help with acid reflux? Unfortunately, there is no easy answer to this question. While it is true that some people find that their symptoms are relieved by eating sweets, for others, sweets can make acid reflux worse. There are a few possible explanations for why sweets might help relieve acid reflux symptoms in some people. One theory is that the sugar in sweets provides a temporary distraction from the pain of acid reflux. Another possibility is that sweets stimulate the production of saliva, which can help to neutralize stomach acids. Whatever the reason, if you find that eating sweets helps to relieve your acid reflux symptoms, there is no need to feel guilty about indulging in a little bit of sugar. Just be sure to keep an eye on your portion sizes, as eating too much sugar can lead to weight gain, which can make acid reflux worse. Of course, if you find that eating sweets makes your acid reflux worse, it's best to avoid them altogether. There are plenty of other delicious foods that won't trigger your symptoms, so you don't need to miss out on the joy of eating just to avoid acid reflux.

What is the symptoms of reflux esophagitis?

There are a few symptoms that are indicative of reflux esophagitis. Perhaps the most obvious symptom is heartburn. This is a burning sensation that is felt in the lower chest area. It is caused by stomach acid backing up into the esophagus. Other symptoms include regurgitation, dysphagia, and chest pain. Regurgitation is when stomach contents are brought back up into the throat. This can happen after a meal or at any time during the day. Dysphagia is when it is difficult to swallow. This may be because of the presence of food or stomach acid in the esophagus. Chest pain is another symptom that is often associated with reflux esophagitis. This pain can vary in intensity and may be felt in the middle or left side of the chest. It is important to see a doctor if you are experiencing any chest pain, as it could also be a sign of a heart attack. These are just some of the symptoms that are associated with reflux esophagitis. If you are experiencing any of these, it is important to see a doctor so that they can properly diagnose and treat the condition.

How do you fix reflux esophagitis?

There are a number of different ways that you can treat reflux esophagitis. The first step is to identify the underlying cause of the condition. Once the cause has been identified, you can start to treat the symptoms. Reflux esophagitis is often caused by a malfunctioning lower esophageal sphincter (LES). The LES is a ring of muscle that separates the stomach from the esophagus. Normally, the LES opens to allow food and liquid to pass into the stomach. Once the food has passed into the stomach, the LES closes to prevent stomach contents from flowing back into the esophagus. If the LES is not working properly, stomach contents can flow back up into the esophagus. This can cause a number of different symptoms, including heartburn, chest pain, and difficulty swallowing. In some cases, reflux esophagitis can also cause bleeding or ulcers in the esophagus. There are a number of different ways to treat reflux esophagitis. The first step is to identify the underlying cause of the condition. Once the cause has been identified, you can start to treat the symptoms. One of the most effective treatments for reflux esophagitis is lifestyle changes. If you are overweight or obese, you can reduce your risk of symptoms by losing weight. If you smoke, quitting smoking can also help to reduce your symptoms. Avoiding trigger foods and eating smaller, more frequent meals can also help to reduce symptoms. In some cases, medications may be necessary to control symptoms. Over-the-counter antacids can help to neutralize stomach acid and provide temporary relief from symptoms. Prescription medications, such as proton pump inhibitors (PPIs) and H2 blockers, can also be effective in treating reflux esophagitis. Surgery is an option for severe cases that do not respond to other treatments. If you are suffering from reflux esophagitis, there are a number of treatment options available. Talk to your doctor about your symptoms and the best course of treatment for you.

How serious is reflux esophagitis?

Acid reflux, also known as gastroesophageal reflux disease (GERD), is a condition in which the contents of the stomach flow back up into the esophagus. This can cause a burning sensation in the chest or throat, known as heartburn. While occasional acid reflux is not a cause for concern, reflux esophagitis is a more serious condition that can lead to nausea, vomiting, and difficulty swallowing. In some cases, reflux esophagitis can cause bleeding or ulcers in the esophagus. If left untreated, reflux esophagitis can lead to a number of complications, such as Barrett's esophagus and esophageal cancer. Therefore, it is important to see a doctor if you experience symptoms of reflux esophagitis, such as heartburn that doesn't go away, difficulty swallowing, or bleeding in the esophagus.

Does reflux esophagitis go away?

Acid reflux, also known as GERD, is a condition where stomach acid backs up into the esophagus. This can cause a burning sensation in the chest or throat, and can sometimes be severe enough to cause trouble breathing. Many people with acid reflux only have mild symptoms, and the condition can be managed with lifestyle changes and over-the-counter medications. However, some people with acid reflux may develop a more serious condition called reflux esophagitis. Reflux esophagitis is a condition in which the lining of the esophagus is inflamed by stomach acid. This can cause a range of symptoms, including heartburn, chest pain, trouble swallowing, and a feeling of something being stuck in the throat. In some cases, reflux esophagitis can lead to bleeding or ulcers in the esophagus. Reflux esophagitis is generally a chronic condition, which means it can last for a long time. There is no cure for reflux esophagitis, but there are treatments that can help to manage the symptoms and keep the condition under control. Medications called proton pump inhibitors (PPIs) can be effective in reducing stomach acid production, and thus relieving symptoms. In some cases, surgery may be necessary to tighten the lower esophageal sphincter (the muscle that separates the stomach from the esophagus), which can help to prevent stomach acid from backing up into the esophagus. Despite treatment, reflux esophagitis may not go away completely, and flare-ups can occur. However, with proper treatment and management, the condition can be controlled and the symptoms kept to a minimum.

What is the most likely cause of the reflux esophagitis?

Acid reflux is a disorder in which the acidic contents of the stomach escape upwards into the throat, causing symptoms such as heartburn and a sour taste in the mouth. The most likely cause of this condition is a failure of the lower esophageal sphincter (LES) to close properly, allowing stomach acids to back up into the esophagus. Other potential causes include eating large meals, lying down immediately after eating, and consuming certain foods or drinks that are known to trigger acid reflux. Treatment for acid reflux typically involves lifestyle changes, such as avoiding trigger foods and eating smaller meals, and may also include medication.

What is the difference between acid reflux and esophagitis?

There are a few key differences between acid reflux and esophagitis. First, acid reflux is a disorder characterized by the backflow of stomach acid into the esophagus. This can cause a variety of symptoms, including heartburn, chest pain, and a sour taste in the mouth. Esophagitis, on the other hand, is an inflammation of the esophagus. This can be caused by a number of things, including acid reflux, infection, or allergic reaction. Esophagitis can cause a variety of symptoms, including pain, difficulty swallowing, and nausea. Acid reflux and esophagitis are both fairly common conditions, and they often occur together. Treatment for both conditions typically includes lifestyle changes, such as eating a healthy diet and avoiding triggering foods, as well as medications to reduce stomach acid production. In some cases, surgery may be necessary to treat esophagitis.

While there is no cure for acid reflux, there are many treatments that can help to reduce the symptoms. Over-the-counter antacids can be taken to help neutralize stomach acid. Prescription medications can be used to reduce the production of stomach acid. In severe cases, surgery may be necessary to repair the damage caused by acid reflux.

What happens if esophagitis is left untreated?

If esophagitis is left untreated, the esophagus can become scarred and narrow. This can make it difficult to swallow and can lead to choking. Esophageal cancer is a rare but serious complication of untreated esophagitis.

How long does reflux esophagitis last?

How long does esophageal reflux last? This is a tough question to answer because it depends on the severity of the reflux and the person's individual response to treatment. In general, though, most people find that their symptoms start to improve within a few weeks of starting treatment. For some people, the symptoms may go away completely. For others, the symptoms may come and go, or they may be more constant but not necessarily severe. There are a number of different factors that can contribute to how long esophageal reflux lasts. One of the most important is the severity of the reflux. People with more severe reflux may find that their symptoms last longer or are more difficult to treat. Another important factor is the person's response to treatment. Some people may find that their symptoms improve quickly with treatment, while others may find that it takes longer for their symptoms to improve. There are a number of different treatments for esophageal reflux, and the type of treatment that is most effective for a person may vary depending on the person's individual situation. In general, though, most people with esophageal reflux will find that lifestyle changes, such as avoiding trigger foods and eating smaller meals, can help to reduce their symptoms. Medications, such as antacids and proton pump inhibitors, can also be effective in treating symptoms of esophageal reflux. In some cases, surgery may be necessary to treat severe cases of esophageal reflux. If you are suffering from symptoms of esophageal reflux, it is important to talk to your doctor so that you can develop a treatment plan that is right for you. with treatment, most people find that their symptoms improve within a few weeks. However, the length of time that it takes for symptoms to improve may vary depending on the severity of the reflux and the person's individual response to treatment.

What foods soothe esophagitis?

Acid reflux, also known as gastroesophageal reflux disease (GERD), is a condition where stomach acid flows back up into the esophagus. This can cause heartburn, chest pain, and other uncomfortable symptoms. There are many different foods that can help ease the symptoms of acid reflux. Some people find that certain foods help to soothe their esophagitis, while others find that certain foods trigger their symptoms. Some of the best foods for relieving acid reflux include: -Oatmeal: This breakfast staple is a great source of fiber and can help to absorb stomach acid. -Almonds: These nuts contain high levels of calcium and can help to neutralize stomach acid. -Ginger: Ginger is a common remedy for gastrointestinal issues and can help to reduce the production of stomach acid. -Yogurt: This probiotic-rich food can help to promote a healthy balance of gut bacteria, which can help to reduce the symptoms of acid reflux. -Green vegetables: Vegetables like spinach and kale are high in fiber and can help to keep the digestive system moving properly, reducing the risk of acid reflux. -Fennel:

This herb has been shown to help reduce the symptoms of acid reflux and can be enjoyed in many ways, such as added to salads or cooked as a side dish. -Chamomile tea: This herbal tea can help to soothe the digestive system and reduce the production of stomach acid. Making lifestyle changes, such as avoiding trigger foods, quitting smoking, and losing weight, can also help to reduce the symptoms of acid reflux. If lifestyle changes and diet modification do not provide relief, medications may be necessary to control the symptoms of acid reflux.

What naturally heals esophagitis?

There is no one-size-fits-all answer to the question of what naturally heals esophagitis. However, some Natural approaches may provide relief, including: -Identifying and avoiding foods and drinks that trigger or worsen symptoms. Common triggers include acidic foods and drinks, such as citrus fruits and juices, tomatoes, chocolate, coffee, and alcoholic beverages. -Eating smaller, more frequent meals and avoiding eating late at night. -Chewing gum or sucking on hard candy to increase saliva production and reduce reflux. - Wearing loose-fitting clothes to avoid added pressure on the stomach. -Losing weight if overweight or obese. -Quitting smoking. -Raising the head of your bed by 6 to 8 inches with blocks under the bedposts. -Avoiding lying down for three hours after eating. - Sleeping on your left side to reduce the risk of nighttime heartburn. If these natural approaches do not provide relief, medications that reduce or block stomach acid may be necessary. These include antacids, H2 blockers, and proton pump inhibitors. Surgery is rarely needed to treat esophagitis.

What does esophagitis pain feel like?

Pain from esophagitis may be constant or may come and go. The pain is often worse when you swallow or bend over. You may feel like food is getting stuck in your throat. The pain may be burning, sharp, or cramping. You may also have hiccups, burp a lot, or get sour taste in your mouth. Your doctor may also call this gastroesophageal reflux disease (GERD) or peptic esophagitis. If you have esophagitis, your esophagus, the tube that goes from your throat to your stomach, is inflamed. This can happen because of: Acid backing up from your stomach Eating large meals or lying down right after eating An infection Certain medicines A chemical, such as lye, going down your throat Esophagitis can happen at any age, but it is more common in adults. Many people with esophagitis also have GERD.

What foods should be avoided with esophagitis?

There are a few different types of esophagitis, all with different dietary triggers and severity. In this article, we will focus on Gastroesophageal Reflux Disease (GERD) and Eosinophilic Esophagitis (EoE), as these are the two most common types of esophagitis. GERD is a chronic condition caused by the backflow of stomach contents and acids into the esophagus. This can cause symptoms like heartburn, chest pain, trouble swallowing, and a sour taste in the mouth. While anyone can experience occasional heartburn after eating spicy or fatty foods, those with GERD experience it more frequently, and it can cause serious damage to the esophagus over time. There are a few things you can do to manage GERD and reduce the likelihood of flare-ups, including avoiding trigger foods. Common trigger foods include: -Citrus fruits and juices -Tomatoes and tomato sauce -Chocolate -Onions -Coffee and tea -Alcohol -Mint -Spicy foods Of course, trigger foods will vary from person to person. You may find that you can eat some of the above foods without any problems, while others will cause serious heartburn. It's important to pay attention to your body and what foods make your symptoms worse. EoE is a less common but equally unpleasant condition. It is caused by an allergic reaction in the esophagus, and symptoms include difficulty swallowing, abdominal pain, heartburn, and vomiting. EoE is often triggered by foods that contain a lot of protein, including: -Beef -Chicken -Fish - Eggs -Nuts -Dairy As with GERD, everyone will have different trigger foods, so it's important to pay attention to your body and what makes your symptoms worse. While avoiding trigger foods is the best way to manage both GERD and EoE, it's not always possible, and some flare-ups are inevitable. If you do experience a flare-up, there are a few things you can do to help ease your symptoms: -Take an over-the-counter antacid -Drink plenty of fluids -Eat smaller, more frequent meals -Avoid tight-fitting clothing -Elevate your head when you sleep

Can you fully recover from esophagitis?

The condition known as esophagitis refers to the inflammation of the esophagus, which is the tube connecting the throat to the stomach. This can be a very painful condition, as the esophagus is constantly being used for swallowing. There are many different causes of esophagitis, but the most common is gastroesophageal reflux disease (GERD). GERD is a condition in which the stomach contents and acids flow back up into the esophagus. This can cause a burning sensation in the chest or throat, and can also lead to difficulty swallowing. Esophagitis can be a very serious condition, and if left untreated, can lead to ulcers, bleeding, and even cancer of the esophagus. However, it is important to note that esophagitis is treatable, and many people are able to fully recover from the condition. The first step in treatment is to identify the underlying cause of the esophagitis and to treat that. For example, if GERD is the cause, then treatment will focus on reducing the amount of acid in the stomach and preventing the reflux of acid into the esophagus. This can be done with medication, diet, and lifestyle changes. In addition, it is important to focus on the symptoms of esophagitis and to treat them accordingly. For example, pain relievers can be used to help with the pain, and antacids can be used to neutralize the stomach acids that are causing the burning sensation. It is also important to eat soft, bland foods and to avoid foods that are acidic or spicy, as these can aggravate the symptoms. With treatment, most people with esophagitis are able to fully recover and live normal, healthy lives. However, it is important to work with a healthcare provider to create a treatment plan that is right for you.

Acid reflux, also known as GERD, is a condition in which the stomach contents leak backward from the stomach into the esophagus. This can cause heartburn, chest pain, and regurgitation. If left untreated, GERD can lead to Barrett's esophagus, which is a precancerous condition. Treatment options for GERD include lifestyle changes, such as avoiding trigger foods and eating smaller meals, and medications, such as antacids and proton pump inhibitors.

Can stress cause esophagitis?

It is commonly believed that stress is a trigger for acid reflux and other gastrointestinal problems. The thinking is that when we are stressed, we produce more stomach acid than normal. This excess stomach acid then leaks out of the stomach and up into the esophagus, causing irritation and pain. However, there is no scientific evidence to support this claim. In fact, some studies have shown that stress may actually protect the stomach from producing too much acid. So, while stress may not be a direct cause of esophagitis, it may contribute to other factors that can lead to the condition. For example, people who are under a lot of stress may be more likely to smoke or drink alcohol. Both of these habits can increase the risk of esophagitis. Stress may also lead to other unhealthy behaviors, such as not eating enough or not getting enough exercise, which can also contribute to the development of esophagitis. If you are struggling with stress, there are many different ways to manage it. Some people find that relaxation techniques, such as yoga or meditation, can help. Others may need to seek counseling or therapy to deal with the underlying issues that are causing their stress. If you think that stress may be a factor in your esophagitis, talk to your doctor. They can help you to identify other potential causes and recommend the best treatment for you.

What are the stages of esophagitis?

There are four main stages of esophagitis: The first stage, called erosive esophagitis, is characterized by small lesions or erosions in the esophageal lining. These erosions can cause bleeding and ulceration. The second stage, called ulcerative esophagitis, is characterized by the development of ulcers in the esophageal lining. These ulcers can bleed and cause pain. The third stage, called stenosis, is characterized by the narrowing of the esophageal lumen. This narrowing can make it difficult to swallow. The fourth stage, called Barrett's esophagus, is characterized by the change of the esophageal lining from stratified squamous epithelium to columnar epithelium. This change is believed to be a precancerous condition.

When should I be concerned about esophagitis?

Acid reflux and esophagitis are usually not serious. However, if you have esophagitis, it is important to find out what is causing it. If left untreated, esophagitis can damage the lining of your esophagus and cause bleeding. You may also be at risk for Barrett's esophagus, which is a precancerous condition. If you have any of the following symptoms, you should see your doctor: -Difficulty swallowing -Weight loss -Anemia -Vomiting blood -Black stools -Chest pain -Difficulty breathing Your doctor will likely want to do an endoscopy to check for damage to your esophagus. During this procedure, a small camera is passed down your throat so that your doctor can look for signs of damage. Your doctor may also recommend a biopsy, which is a procedure in which a small sample of tissue is taken from your esophagus for further testing. If you have esophagitis, there are several treatments that can help. Antacids and other medications can help to reduce stomach acid. Surgery may be an option in severe cases. If you have esophagitis, it is important to follow your doctor's instructions and to make lifestyle changes, such as avoiding trigger foods and eating smaller meals. With treatment, esophagitis can usually be cured.

Is banana good for esophagitis?

Banana is known to be a godsend for those suffering from heartburn and indigestion, but what about esophagitis? This condition is a bit more serious, as it involves inflammation of the esophagus lining, and can cause pain, difficulty swallowing, and nausea. There are a few different types of esophagitis, and the treatment depends on the underlying cause. However, diet plays an important role in managing the condition and maintaining good esophageal health. So, let's take a closer look at whether banana is good for esophagitis. As mentioned, diet is vitally important for those suffering from esophagitis. That's because what you eat can either aggravate the condition or help to ease symptoms. So, it's important to choose your foods carefully. Generally speaking, foods that are soft, bland, and easy to digest are best. That's because these types of foods are less likely to irritate the inflamed lining of the esophagus. Banana fits into this category, as it's a soft fruit that is easy to digest. In fact, banana is often recommended as a dietary option for those with digestive issues. Additionally, banana contains a type of fibre known as pectin. This soluble fibre helps to absorb water and form a gel-like substance, which can coating the lining of the esophagus and protect it from irritation. So, all in all, banana is a good option for those suffering from esophagitis. It's a soft, bland food that is easy to digest and contains a type of fibre that can help to protect the esophageal lining.

How did I get esophagitis?

There are many things that can contribute to someone getting esophagitis. Some of the most common reasons are due to acid reflux or GERD. Other contributing factors can be from other medical conditions, treatments, or infections. Acid reflux occurs when stomach acid backs up into the esophagus. This happens when the lower esophageal sphincter (LES) muscle relaxes more often than it should or is not able to close properly. This allows gastric contents and acid to rise up into the esophagus, irritating the lining. There are a variety of other medical conditions that can also lead to esophagitis. These can include: - Hiatal hernia: This occurs when the opening in the diaphragm that the esophagus goes through is too large. This can cause the LES to open more often, leading to acid reflux. - Scleroderma: This is a condition that causes the hardening and tightening of the skin and connective tissues. This can also lead to a weakening of the LES, resulting in acid reflux. - Peptic ulcer disease: This is a condition where sores form in the lining of the stomach or small intestine. The ulcers can erode the esophageal lining, leading to esophagitis. There are also a number of treatments that can contribute to esophagitis. These include: - Radiation therapy: This treatment can damage the esophageal lining, leading to esophagitis. - Certain medications: There are a number of medications that can irritate the esophageal lining, including some antibiotics, pain relievers, and bisphosphonates (used to treat osteoporosis). Additionally, there are a few infections that can cause esophagitis. The most common of these is candidiasis, which is a fungal infection. Other infections that can cause esophagitis include: - Herpes simplex virus - Cytomegalovirus - Human papillomavirus Esophagitis can be a very painful condition. It is important to see a doctor if you think you may be suffering from esophagitis so that they can properly diagnose and treat the condition.

Does esophagitis come on suddenly?

There are many things that can cause sudden onset esophagitis. It could be a reaction to a medication, an infection, or even just a change in your diet. However, it is also important to remember that not every case of esophagitis comes on suddenly. Sometimes, it can develop gradually over time. If you think you may have esophagitis, it is important to see a doctor right away. Esophagitis can cause serious problems if it is not treated, such as bleeding or difficulty swallowing. If you are experiencing any symptoms of esophagitis, such as pain or difficulty swallowing, contact your doctor immediately.

Why do I keep getting esophagitis?

If you are suffering from persistent esophagitis, it is important to speak to your doctor to rule out any potential underlying causes. Common causes of esophagitis include gastroesophageal reflux disease (GERD), postnasal drip, viral infections, and, rarely, certain medications. GERD is a chronic digestive disorder that occurs when stomach contents wash back up into the esophagus. This acidic backwash can irritate the lining of the esophagus and lead to esophagitis. In addition to esophagitis, GERD can also cause heartburn, coughing, and chest pain. Postnasal drip occurs when excessive mucus drains from the sinuses into the back of the throat. This can happen when you have a cold, the flu, or allergies. The excess mucus can irritate the lining of the esophagus and lead to esophagitis. Viral infections are a common cause of esophagitis. The viruses that most commonly cause esophagitis include the herpes simplex virus (HSV), the varicella-zoster virus (VZV), and the cytomegalovirus (CMV). Esophagitis caused by HSV is usually the most severe, and can lead to ulcers and scarring of the esophagus. CMV esophagitis is less common, but can be serious in people with weakened immune systems. Certain medications can also cause esophagitis. The most common offenders are nonsteroidal anti-inflammatory drugs (NSAIDs), such as ibuprofen and naproxen. These medications can irritate the esophagus and lead to inflammation. Other medications that can cause esophagitis include bisphosphonates, potassium products, quinidine, and doxycycline. If you are experiencing any symptoms of esophagitis, it is important to see your doctor. Esophagitis can be a painful and debilitating condition, but it is often treatable. With the help of your doctor, you can find the underlying cause of your esophagitis and get the treatment you need to feel better.

While there is no cure for acid reflux, there are treatments that can help to relieve the symptoms. Avoiding trigger foods, eating smaller meals, and avoiding eating late at night can help to prevent acid reflux episodes. Over-the-counter antacids can also help to neutralize stomach acid and provide relief. If symptoms persist, it is important to see a doctor, as acid reflux can lead to more serious conditions such as GERD.

How do you confirm esophagitis?

Esophagitis is a condition in which the esophagus, the muscular tube that connects the mouth to the stomach, becomes inflamed. This inflammation can be caused by a number of things, including stomach acid and certain medications. Esophagitis can lead to a number of symptoms, including heartburn, chest pain, difficulty swallowing, and nausea. If you think you might have esophagitis, it's important to see your doctor for a proper diagnosis. They will likely start by asking about your symptoms and medical history. They will also likely perform a physical exam. In some cases, they may also order tests, such as an endoscopy or biopsy. An endoscopy is a procedure in which a thin, flexible tube with a camera is inserted down the throat and into the esophagus. This allows the doctor to get a close look at the inside of the esophagus and look for signs of inflammation.

A biopsy is a procedure in which a small sample of tissue is taken from the esophagus and examined in a laboratory. This can help confirm the diagnosis of esophagitis. If you have esophagitis, it's important to work with your doctor to find a treatment that works for you. Treatment will likely focus on relieving the symptoms and healing the inflammation. This may involve lifestyle changes, such as avoiding trigger foods and quitting smoking. Medications, such as proton pump inhibitors and antacids, may also be used. In some cases, surgery may be necessary.

Do you feel sick with esophagitis?

If you have esophagitis, you may feel sick. This is because esophagitis is an inflammation of the esophagus, which is the tube that carries food from your mouth to your stomach. When this tube is inflamed, it can cause a feeling of sickness. Esophagitis can also cause other symptoms, such as pain when you swallow, heartburn, and chest pain. If you have esophagitis, it is important to see your doctor. Esophagitis is a serious condition and can lead to other health problems, such as ulcers, bleeding, and scarring of the esophagus. If esophagitis is not treated, it can make it difficult to swallow, and you may lose weight. Esophagitis is usually treated with medication. Medications used to treat esophagitis include antacids, H2 blockers, and proton pump inhibitors. These medications can help to reduce the inflammation and pain associated with esophagitis. In some cases, surgery may be necessary to treat esophagitis. If you have esophagitis, there are some things you can do to help improve your symptoms. Avoiding foods that trigger your symptoms, such as spicy or acidic foods, can help to reduce the pain and inflammation associated with esophagitis. Eating small meals, and avoiding foods that are difficult to swallow, can also help. Quitting smoking can also help to reduce the symptoms of esophagitis. Esophagitis is a serious condition that can cause a great deal of pain and discomfort. If you think you may have esophagitis, it is important to see your doctor so that you can get the treatment you need. There are many treatments available for esophagitis, and with the proper treatment, you can find relief from your symptoms and improve your quality of life.

Is esophagitis cancerous?

The Human Esophagus The esophagus is a long, hollow tube that runs from the throat to the stomach. It is about 10 inches long and is lined with a moist, pink tissue called mucosa. The esophagus serves two main purposes: to move food from the throat to the stomach, and to keep food from returning back up from the stomach to the throat. The esophagus is made up of several layers of tissue. The innermost layer is called the mucosa. The mucosa contains many small blood vessels and is lined with tiny, finger-like projections called villi. The villi absorb nutrients from the food we eat and help move it through the digestive system. The next layer is the submucosa. The submucosa contains blood vessels, lymph vessels, and nerve fibers. These structures help to keep the mucosa healthy and provide nutrients for the tissue. The third and final layer is the muscle layer. The muscle layer consists of two types of muscles: smooth muscles and skeletal muscles. The smooth muscles are responsible for moving food through the esophagus and keep the opening between the esophagus and stomach closed. The skeletal muscles help to move the esophagus when we swallow. The esophagus is a very strong and flexible tube. It is able to expand when we eat and drink and then return to its normal size. The esophagus is able to do this because of the muscle layer. The muscle layer is made up of two types of muscles: smooth muscles and skeletal muscles. The smooth muscles are responsible for moving food through the esophagus and keep the opening between the esophagus and stomach closed. The skeletal muscles help to move the esophagus when we swallow. Swallowing is a complex process that is controlled by both voluntary and involuntary muscle movements. When we see food or drink, our brain sends a signal to our muscles to start the process of swallowing. The muscles in our throat and mouth begin to contract and push the food or drink towards the back of our throat. At the same time, the muscles in our esophagus begin to contract and push the food or drink down towards our stomach. Once the food or drink enters the esophagus, it is moved along by a series of rhythmic muscle contractions called peristalsis. Peristalsis is an involuntary muscle movement that propels the contents of our gastrointestinal tract forwards. The esophagus is able to move food or drink downwards because it is lined with a layer of slippery mucus. This mucus lubricates the food or drink and prevents it from sticking to the esophageal walls. The esophagus is a very strong and flexible tube. It is able to expand when we eat and drink and then return to its normal size. The esophagus is able to do this because of the muscle layer. The muscle layer is made

Do I need an endoscopy for acid reflux?

Acid reflux is a condition in which stomach acid flows back up into the esophagus, causing symptoms like heartburn, nausea, and sore throat. While occasional acid reflux is nothing to worry about, persistent acid reflux may be a sign of a more serious condition called gastroesophageal reflux disease (GERD). GERD is a chronic form of acid reflux that can cause damage to the esophagus if left untreated. While most people with GERD manage their symptoms with lifestyle changes and over-the-counter medications, some people may require prescription medications or surgery. Endoscopy is a procedure that allows your doctor to visualize the inside of your esophagus and stomach. This test is generally reserved for people with persistent or severe symptoms of acid reflux. During an endoscopy, your doctor will insert a small, flexible tube with a camera attached into your mouth and down your throat. The camera will provide your doctor with a clear view of the inside of your esophagus and stomach. If your doctor sees any damage to the esophageal lining, they may biopsy (take a small sample of) the tissue to be analyzed in a laboratory. Your doctor may recommend an endoscopy if you have persistent symptoms of acid reflux that are not relieved by lifestyle changes or over-the-counter medications. They may also recommend this test if you have any symptoms of GERD, such as trouble swallowing, weight loss, or bleeding. If you have been experiencing symptoms of acid reflux, speak to your doctor to see if an endoscopy is right for you.

What can make esophagitis worse?

There are various factors that can make esophagitis worse. Some of these include: - Eating large meals - Eating high-fat foods - Drinking alcohol - Smoking - Being overweight or obese - Wearing tight-fitting clothes - Having a hiatal hernia - Eating late at night Eating large meals can put extra pressure on the lower esophageal sphincter (LES), which can cause it to open and allow stomach acids to reflux back up into the esophagus. Eating high-fat foods can also trigger symptoms, as Fat takes longer to digest so it spends more time in the stomach, providing more opportunity for acids to reflux. Alcohol relaxes the LES, Smoking cessation can be difficult, but it is worth it as tobacco use is a major risk factor for esophageal cancer. Being overweight or obese can also increase the risk of reflux, as there is more pressure on the LES. Wearing tight-fitting clothes can also exacerbate symptoms, as it puts pressure on the stomach and can cause the LES to open. Having a hiatal hernia, where the stomach protrudes through the diaphragm, can also cause reflux as it can weaken the LES. Eating late at night can trigger symptoms as well, as lying down after a meal can allow acids to reflux more easily. There are various things that can make esophagitis worse, and it is important to be aware of these triggers in order to minimize the risk of symptoms.

Does milk help esophagitis?

The question of whether milk helps esophagitis is a complicated one. Esophagitis is a condition in which the esophagus, the tube that carries food from the mouth to the stomach, becomes inflamed. This can be caused by a number of things, including gastroesophageal reflux disease (GERD), certain medications, and certain medical procedures. GERD is a condition in which stomach acid flows back up into the esophagus, causing inflammation. This can happen if the valve between the stomach and the esophagus is not working properly. certain medications, such as NSAIDs, can also cause esophagitis. And, finally, certain medical procedures, such as endoscopy, can also cause the condition. So, does milk help esophagitis? The answer is, it depends. Milk can help to soothe the esophagus and make the symptoms of esophagitis less severe. However, it is important to remember that milk is also a source of fat and calories. For people who are struggling with esophagitis, consuming too much milk can actually make the condition worse. If you are struggling with esophagitis, it is important to talk to your doctor about the best way to manage your condition. They may recommend a specific diet plan, or they may prescribe medication to help control the symptoms.

How do you treat esophagitis at home?

Acid reflux, also known as gastroesophageal reflux disease (GERD), is a condition in which the contents of your stomach reflux or "back up" into your esophagus. This can cause a burning sensation in your chest or throat, and can, over time, damage your esophagus. There are a few things you can do at home to help relieve your symptoms and prevent further damage to your esophagus. First, try to identify your triggers. Common triggers include fatty or fried foods, spicy foods, chocolate, mint, caffeine, alcohol, and smoking. Avoiding these triggers can help reduce the frequency and severity of your symptoms. Second, eat small meals. Eating smaller meals more frequently can help lessen the amount of stomach acid that enters your esophagus. Third, eat slowly and chew your food thoroughly. This gives your stomach time to properly digest your food and also reduces the risk of regurgitation. Fourth, try to maintain a healthy weight. Excess weight can put additional pressure on your stomach, which can lead to reflux. Finally, sleep with your head elevated. This can help reduce the amount of stomach acid that enters your esophagus while you are asleep. If you are experiencing symptoms of acid reflux, or esophagitis, talk to your doctor. They can help you create a plan to manage your symptoms and prevent further damage to your esophagus.

Acid reflux can be a painful and dangerous condition if left untreated. However, with proper diagnosis and treatment, most people with acid reflux can live relatively normal and healthy lives. If you think you may be suffering from acid reflux, be sure to see your doctor for proper diagnosis and treatment.

What is the best drink for esophagitis?

There are a few different drinks that can help ease the symptoms of esophagitis. Peppermint tea is a great option because it can help to soothe the stomach and relax the muscles in the digestive tract. Chamomile tea is another good choice because it is an anti-inflammatory agent. Ginger root tea is also beneficial because it can help to reduce nausea. There are also a few different types of juice that can be helpful, such as aloe vera juice and cucumber juice.

What drinks help heal the esophagus?

There are a few different things that you can drink that will help heal your esophagus from acid reflux. Water is always a great choice and will help to keep your throat and esophagus lubricated. You can also drink herbal teas that will help soothe the area and calm the stomach. Some good choices are ginger tea, chamomile tea, or licorice tea. You can also try drinking some clear soups or broth to help with the healing process.

Does esophagitis go away without treatment?

It is not clear how often esophagitis goes away without treatment. In general, the outlook for people with esophagitis is good. Most people with the condition improve within a few weeks of beginning treatment. However, some people may have recurrent bouts of esophagitis, especially if they do not receive long-term treatment or do not follow their doctor's recommendations for managing the condition. Esophagitis can also lead to complications, such as narrowing of the esophagus (esophageal stricture) or bleeding. These complications can be serious and, in rare cases, life-threatening.

How long can you live if you have Barrett's esophagus?

Barrett's esophagus is a condition in which the tissue lining the esophagus changes, becoming more like the tissue lining the intestine. This change is thought to be a result of longstanding acid reflux. Barrett's esophagus is considered a precancerous condition because it increases the risk of esophageal cancer. The good news is that Barrett's esophagus can be detected early and treated. In most cases, Barrett's esophagus does not-Progress to cancer. In fact, with early diagnosis and proper treatment, the vast majority of people with Barrett's esophagus will never develop esophageal cancer. Still, it's important to be aware of the risks associated with Barrett's esophagus and to see your doctor for regular check-ups. If you have Barrett's esophagus, you'll need to have endoscopies more frequently than people without the condition. An endoscopy is a procedure in which a lighted tube is used to examine the inside of the esophagus. If you have Barrett's esophagus, you can take steps to reduce your risk of developing esophageal cancer. quit smoking, avoid Barrett's triggers (such as fatty foods and caffeine), and take medication to control GERD.

Can Barrett's esophagus be cured?

Barrett's esophagus is a condition in which the tissue lining the esophagus changes, becoming more like the tissue that lines the intestine. This change is thought to be in response to chronic exposure to stomach acid. Barrett's esophagus is considered a precancerous condition because it increases the risk of developing esophageal cancer. Although there is no cure for Barrett's esophagus, there are treatments that can help to prevent the progression to cancer. These treatments include medications to reduce stomach acid and surgery to remove the damaged tissue. In some cases, ablation (destruction) of the Barrett's tissue can be performed using radiofrequency waves or lasers. If you have Barrett's esophagus, it is important to be monitored by a physician so that any changes in the tissue can be detected early. Early detection and treatment of Barrett's esophagus can significantly reduce the risk of developing esophageal cancer.

How long does it take for Barrett's esophagus to turn to cancer?

Barrett's esophagus is a condition in which the tissue lining the esophagus becomes damaged, usually as a result of acid reflux. Over time, this damage can lead to precancerous changes in the esophagus, which can eventually lead to cancer. While the exact timeline from Barrett's esophagus to cancer is not known, studies have shown that it can take anywhere from several years to several decades. In fact, many people with Barrett's esophagus never develop cancer, and the condition is often only discovered when the person undergoes testing for another reason. However, it is important to be aware of the potential risks associated with Barrett's esophagus, and to see a doctor if you experience any symptoms of the condition, such as GERD, heartburn, or trouble swallowing. If you have Barrett's esophagus, your doctor will likely recommend regular screenings to check for precancerous changes, and may recommend treatment to prevent the progression to cancer.

What is the main cause of Barrett's esophagus?

Barrett's esophagus is a condition in which the tissue lining the esophagus changes, becoming more like the tissue lining the intestines. This change is often, but not always, caused by acid reflux. Acid reflux occurs when stomach acid flows back up into the esophagus. The esophagus is the tube that carries food from the mouth to the stomach. When stomach acid flows back up into the esophagus, it can cause a burning sensation in the chest or throat. This is called heartburn. Heartburn is the most common symptom of Barrett's esophagus. Other symptoms may include: - Regurgitation (the feeling of acid or food coming back up into the throat or mouth) - Chest pain - Difficulty swallowing - A hoarse voice - Coughing People with Barrett's esophagus are at increased risk for esophageal cancer. Esophageal cancer is a cancer that forms in the esophagus. Barrett's esophagus does not cause esophageal cancer, but having Barrett's esophagus increases the risk for developing esophageal cancer. People with Barrett's esophagus should see a doctor for regular check-ups. During these check-ups, the doctor will look for changes in the esophagus. People with Barrett's esophagus may need to have a biopsy. A biopsy is a procedure in which a small piece of tissue is removed from the esophagus and examined under a microscope. Barrett's esophagus can be treated, but it cannot be cured. Treatment options include: - Medications: Medications can be used to treat the symptoms of Barrett's esophagus and to decrease the amount of acid produced by the stomach. - Surgery: Surgery may be an option for people with Barrett's esophagus who are at high risk for esophageal cancer. Surgery is not a cure for Barrett's esophagus, but it may prevent cancer from developing.

Despite its name, acid reflux doesn't involve the stomach. Instead, it is a condition in which the contents of the stomach flow back up the esophagus (the tube that connects the throat to the stomach). This can cause a burning sensation in the chest or throat. Acid reflux is a common condition that can be treated with lifestyle changes and medication.

Should I worry if I have Barrett's esophagus?

Barrett's esophagus is a condition in which the cells lining the esophagus change, becoming more like the cells lining the intestine. This change is thought to be a reaction to damage from stomach acid. People with Barrett's esophagus are at increased risk for developing esophageal cancer. Most people with Barrett's esophagus do not have any symptoms. When symptoms do occur, they may include heartburn, trouble swallowing, or chest pain. These symptoms are also common in other conditions, so they alone are not enough to diagnose Barrett's esophagus. Diagnosis of Barrett's esophagus is usually made through an endoscopy, a procedure in which a flexible tube is inserted through the mouth and into the esophagus. During the endoscopy, a biopsy (a small sample of tissue) is taken from the esophagus. The tissue is then examined under a microscope to look for the changes that are characteristic of Barrett's esophagus. Barrett's esophagus can be found in a small percentage of the general population (estimates range from 0.5% to 3%). The condition is more common in men than in women and is more likely to occur in people over the age of 50.

People with Barrett's esophagus are also more likely to have a family history of the condition. The risk of developing esophageal cancer is thought to be higher in people with Barrett's esophagus, although the absolute risk is still relatively low. Estimates of the risk range from 0.5% to 3% over the course of a lifetime. The risk is thought to be highest in people with Barrett's esophagus that is associated with certain other factors, such as intestinal metaplasia (a condition in which the cells lining the esophagus change, becoming more like the cells lining the intestine) and a high number of esophageal squamous cells. While the risk of esophageal cancer is higher in people with Barrett's esophagus, it is important to remember that the absolute risk is still relatively low. For most people with Barrett's esophagus, the condition will not progress to cancer. There are several treatment options for Barrett's esophagus. The goal of treatment is to prevent progression to esophageal cancer. The most common treatment is medication to reduce stomach acid. This can be done with over-the-counter medications, such as antacids, or with prescription medications, such as proton pump inhibitors (PPIs) or histamine2-receptor antagonists (H2RAs). Other treatments for Barrett's esophagus include endoscopic techniques, such as photodynamic therapy (PDT) or endoscopic mucosal resection (EMR), and surgery. PDT involves the use of a light-sensitive medication that is activated by a specific wavelength of light. The light

What are the four stages of Barrett's esophagus?

Barrett's esophagus is a condition in which the normal lining of the esophagus is replaced by tissue that is similar to the lining of the intestine. This condition is thought to be caused by repeated exposure of the esophagus to stomach acid. Over time, this exposure can lead to changes in the cells of the esophagus that can eventually lead to cancer. The four stages of Barrett's esophagus are: 1. Columnar metaplasia: This is the earliest stage of Barrett's esophagus, and is characterized by the replacement of the normal squamous cells that line the esophagus with columnar cells. 2. Low-grade dysplasia: In this stage, there are abnormal changes in the cells that line the esophagus, but these changes are not yet cancerous. 3. High-grade dysplasia: This is the most advanced stage of Barrett's esophagus, and is characterized by the presence of cancerous cells in the esophageal lining. 4. Esophageal adenocarcinoma: This is the final stage of Barrett's esophagus, and is characterized by the presence of a malignant tumor in the esophageal lining.

What foods to avoid with barretts?

Acid reflux is a condition that affects the lower esophageal sphincter (LES), the muscular ring located between the stomach and the esophagus. The LES is responsible for keeping the contents of the stomach in the stomach, where they are meant to be. However, in people with acid reflux, the LES doesn't function properly, allowing stomach contents to flow back up into the esophagus. There are a number of factors that can contribute to acid reflux, including obesity, pregnancy, hiatal hernia, and certain medications. But one of the most important things to keep in mind when trying to prevent acid reflux is what you eat. There are certain foods that can trigger acid reflux, and it's important to be aware of them so you can avoid them. Some common trigger foods include spicy foods, fatty foods, tomatoes, citrus fruits, garlic, chocolate, and mint. These foods can relax the LES or increase the production of acid in the stomach, both of which can lead to acid reflux. Other foods to avoid include carbonated beverages, caffeine, alcohol, and fried foods. If you suffer from acid reflux, it's important to make changes to your diet to help prevent the condition. Avoiding trigger foods is a good place to start, but you may also need to eat smaller meals more frequently throughout the day and avoid eating late at night. Eating a healthy diet, maintaining a healthy weight, and avoiding tobacco products can also help prevent acid reflux.

What is the best drink for Barrett's esophagus?

Barrett's esophagus is a condition that can develop as a result of acid reflux. In Barrett's esophagus, the tissue lining the esophagus is replaced by tissue that is similar to the lining of the intestine. This can lead to serious complications, including cancer of the esophagus. There is no one best drink for Barrett's esophagus, but it is important to avoid beverages that can trigger or worsen acid reflux. These include alcoholic beverages, carbonated beverages, coffee, and tea. Instead, choose non-alcoholic beverages such as water, herbal tea, and low-fat milk. You should also avoid eating large meals and eating late at night. Eating smaller meals more frequently throughout the day can help to reduce the risk of acid reflux.

What is the best treatment for Barrett's esophagus?

Barrett's esophagus is a condition in which the lining of the esophagus is damaged, usually as a result of acid reflux. The damage to the esophagus can lead to a number of problems, including difficulty swallowing, bleeding, and an increased risk of cancer of the esophagus. There is no one best treatment for Barrett's esophagus, as the best approach depends on the individual situation. In some cases, medication may be all that is necessary to control the symptoms of Barrett's esophagus and prevent further damage to the esophagus. In other cases, surgery may be necessary to remove damaged tissue or to treat other complications. Barrett's esophagus is a serious condition that requires close monitoring by a doctor. If you think you may have Barrett's esophagus, or if you have been diagnosed with the condition, it is important to see your doctor for regular check-ups and to discuss the best treatment options for you.

What is the average age for Barrett's esophagus?

The average age for Barrett's esophagus is 50-60 years old. Barrett's esophagus is a condition in which the lining of the esophagus is damaged, usually from stomach acid. This damage can lead to changes in the cells of the esophagus, which can eventually lead to cancer. While Barrett's esophagus is more common in people over the age of 50, it can occur at any age.

Can you stop Barrett's esophagus from progressing?

Barrett's esophagus is a condition in which the cells lining the esophagus change, becoming more like the cells lining the intestine. This change is thought to be caused by repeated exposure to stomach acid. Barrett's esophagus is considered a precancerous condition because it increases the risk of esophageal cancer. There is no sure way to prevent Barrett's esophagus from developing. However, you can reduce your risk by avoiding things that can damage the lining of the esophagus, such as gastroesophageal reflux disease (GERD). GERD is a condition in which stomach acid regularly backs up into the esophagus. This backflow of acid can damage the lining of the esophagus, making it more likely for Barrett's esophagus to develop. There are a few things you can do to reduce your risk of GERD and, in turn, Barrett's esophagus. First, avoid foods and beverages that trigger your GERD symptoms. Common triggers include fatty or fried foods, tomatoes, citrus fruits, chocolate, caffeine, and alcohol. Second, eat smaller meals and avoid eating close to bedtime. Third, lose weight if you are overweight or obese. And fourth, prop your head up with pillows when you sleep to keep stomach acid from flowing back into the esophagus. If you have Barrett's esophagus, there are things you can do to prevent it from progressing to cancer. First, see your doctor regularly for esophageal cancer screenings. During these screenings, your doctor will look for abnormal cell changes in the esophagus. Second, if you smoke, quit smoking. Smoking is a major risk factor for esophageal cancer. Third, avoid damage to the esophagus. This means avoiding GERD and other things that can damage the esophagus, such as regular use of NSAIDs (non-steroidal anti-inflammatory drugs). Barrett's esophagus is a serious condition, but it is important to remember that it is treatable and beatable. By following the above advice, you can greatly reduce your risk of developing esophageal cancer.

Acid reflux, also known as gastroesophageal reflux disease (GERD), can be a painful and irritating condition. The good news is that there are treatments available that can help to reduce the symptoms. If you think you may be suffering from acid reflux, it's important to see a doctor so that they can diagnose and treat the condition.

What is the new treatment for Barrett's esophagus?

Barrett's esophagus is a condition in which the tissue lining the esophagus, the tube that carries food from the mouth to the stomach, becomes damaged. This damage is usually caused by acid reflux, a condition in which stomach acid flows back up into the esophagus. Over time, the damage to the esophagus can lead to cancer of the esophagus. The new treatment for Barrett's esophagus is called endoscopic mucosal resection (EMR). EMR is a procedure in which the damaged tissue lining the esophagus is removed. The doctor uses a special instrument, called an endoscope, to see inside the esophagus and remove the damaged tissue. EMR is often used to treat early stages of Barrett's esophagus. EMR is generally safe and effective, but it is a relatively new procedure, so there is not a lot of long-term data available. The most common side effects of EMR are bleeding and perforation (holes) in the esophagus. These side effects are usually mild and resolve on their own. If you have Barrett's esophagus, talk to your doctor about whether EMR is right for you.

How does Barrett's esophagus feel?

Barrett's esophagus is a condition in which the tissue lining the esophagus changes, becoming more like the tissue lining the intestine. This condition can be caused by persistent acid reflux. Symptoms of Barrett's esophagus may include: heartburn, acid reflux, trouble swallowing, or chest pain. However, many people with Barrett's esophagus do not have any symptoms. If you have Barrett's esophagus, you may be at increased risk for developing esophageal cancer. However, not all people with Barrett's esophagus will develop cancer. If you are experiencing any symptoms of Barrett's esophagus, it is important to see your doctor for a diagnosis.

Is Barrett's esophagus fatal?

Barrett's esophagus is a condition in which the tissue lining the esophagus changes, becoming more like the tissue lining the intestine. This condition is often associated with GERD (gastroesophageal reflux disease). While Barrett's esophagus itself is not fatal, it can increase the risk of developing a type of esophageal cancer called adenocarcinoma. Adenocarcinoma of the esophagus is a rare but aggressive type of cancer. The symptoms of Barrett's esophagus, such as heartburn and indigestion, are also common symptoms of adenocarcinoma. This makes it difficult to detect early. When caught early, adenocarcinoma of the esophagus can be treated with surgery, radiation, and/or chemotherapy. The survival rate for those with early-stage disease is about 50-60%. However, the survival rate for those with late-stage disease is only about 20%. Barrett's esophagus can be a serious condition, but it is important to remember that it is not fatal. With early detection and treatment, the prognosis is good.

What foods help heal the esophagus?

If you suffer from acid reflux, you know how frustrating the condition can be. Between the heartburn, the regurgitation, and the GERD-like symptoms, it's enough to make anyone want to give up on eating altogether. But giving up food isn't an option, and luckily there are certain foods that can help heal the esophagus and make acid reflux less painful. Here are some of the best: 1. Aloe vera Aloe vera is a natural anti-inflammatory, so it can help to soothe the irritation caused by acid reflux. You can find aloe vera juice at most health food stores, or you can grow your own plant to have on hand. 2. Bananas Bananas are a great source of potassium, which can help to neutralize stomach acid. Eat a banana or two every day, or try adding them to smoothies or yogurt. 3. Baby carrots Raw carrots are a great snack for keeping acid reflux at bay. The fiber in the carrots will help to absorb stomach acid, and the low sugar content means they won't trigger any reflux. 4. Ginger Ginger is another natural anti-inflammatory, and it's also great for calming an upset stomach. You can eat ginger in candy form, or add it to sauces or soups. 5. Oatmeal Oatmeal is a bland food that can help to soothe the stomach and absorb stomach acid. It's also a good source of fiber, which can help with constipation, another common symptom of acid reflux. 6. Green leafy vegetables Green leafy vegetables like spinach and kale are packed with nutrients that can help heal the esophagus. They're also low in acid, so they won't trigger any reflux. 7. Greek yogurt Greek yogurt is a great source of protein and calcium, both of which are good for the esophagus. The probiotics in yogurt can also help to improve digestion. 8. Almond milk Almond milk is a great alternative to cow's milk for people with acid reflux. It's high in calcium and low in acid, and it's also a good source of healthy fats. 9. Salmon Salmon is a great source of omega-3 fatty acids, which have anti-inflammatory properties. Salmon is also a good source of protein, which can help to repair the esophageal lining. 10. Chicken Chicken is another good source of protein, and it's a lean meat that won't aggravate acid reflux. You can eat chicken in a variety of

Where do you feel pain with Barrett's esophagus?

The most common symptom associated with Barrett's esophagus is heartburn, which is also known as acid reflux. Heartburn occurs when stomach acid backs up into the esophagus, the tube that carries food from the mouth to the stomach. This backup of stomach acid can cause a burning sensation in the chest. Other symptoms of Barrett's esophagus include: - Chest pain - Difficulty swallowing - Regurgitation - coughing - Wheezing Some people with Barrett's esophagus may not have any symptoms. However, if left untreated, Barrett's esophagus can lead to a serious condition called esophageal cancer. Esophageal cancer is a cancer of the esophagus, the tube that carries food from the mouth to the stomach. Esophageal cancer is a rare but serious condition that can be fatal. If you have any of the symptoms of Barrett's esophagus, it is important to see your doctor. Your doctor will likely perform a physical exam and order some tests. A common test used to diagnose Barrett's esophagus is an endoscopy. An endoscopy is a procedure in which a lighted tube is inserted down the throat. The doctor can then see the esophagus and take a biopsy, a small sample of tissue. Treatment for Barrett's esophagus usually involves changes in diet and lifestyle. These changes can help to reduce symptoms and prevent complications. Medications may also be prescribed to help reduce stomach acid. In some cases, surgery may be necessary.

How fast does Barrett's esophagus progress?

Barrett's esophagus is a condition in which the tissue lining the esophagus is replaced by tissue that is similar to the lining of the intestine. This condition can be caused by gastroesophageal reflux disease (GERD). GERD is a condition in which the contents of the stomach reflux (back up) into the esophagus. The progression of Barrett's esophagus is not well understood. It is thought that the condition progresses slowly over many years. In some cases, Barrett's esophagus may lead to esophageal cancer. Esophageal cancer is a serious, life-threatening condition. There is no sure way to prevent Barrett's esophagus. However, you can help prevent GERD by avoiding foods and beverages that trigger your symptoms, eating small meals, and not eating close to bedtime. You should also avoid tobacco and alcohol. If you have GERD, treatment can help prevent Barrett's esophagus. Treatment options include medications and surgery. If you have Barrett's esophagus, it is important to see your doctor for regular follow-up visits. During these visits, your doctor will perform a endoscopy to check for changes in the lining of your esophagus. If changes are found, a biopsy may be done to check for cancer.

Can damage from Barrett's esophagus be reversed?

Barrett's esophagus is a condition in which the tissue lining the esophagus is replaced by tissue that is similar to the lining of the intestine. This change in the lining of the esophagus is thought to be a result of damage from acid reflux. Acid reflux is a condition in which the stomach contents are forced back up into the esophagus. The stomach contents are highly acidic, and this can damage the lining of the esophagus. It is not clear if the damage from Barrett's esophagus can be reversed. There is some evidence that the damage may be reversible if the condition is caught early and treated with medication. There is also some evidence that the damage may be irreversible if the condition is not treated. If you have Barrett's esophagus, it is important to talk to your doctor about your treatment options. There is no one-size-fits-all treatment for Barrett's esophagus, and the best course of treatment will depend on the individual case.

Acid reflux is a problem that can be remedied with lifestyle changes, over-the-counter medications, and prescription medications. With proper treatment, most people with acid reflux can get relief from their symptoms.

How often should you have an endoscopy if you have Barrett's esophagus?

If you have Barrett's esophagus, you should have an endoscopy every three to five years. This is because people with Barrett's are at an increased risk for developing esophageal cancer. While the chances of developing cancer are still relatively low, it's important to catch it early if it does occur.

How painful is Barrett's esophagus?

Barrett's esophagus is a condition in which the tissue lining the esophagus, the tube that carries food from the throat to the stomach, is replaced by tissue that is similar to the lining of the intestine. This condition is often caused by acid reflux, which is when stomach acid flows back up into the esophagus. Symptoms of Barrett's esophagus may include heartburn, chest pain, and trouble swallowing. The condition can also lead to esophageal cancer. Barrett's esophagus is not usually painful. However, some people may experience discomfort or pain, especially when swallowing. If you experience any pain or discomfort, it is important to talk to your doctor.

Can I drink milk with Barrett's esophagus?

Barrett's esophagus is a condition in which the lining of the esophagus changes, becoming more like the lining of the intestine. This change is thought to be due to chronic irritation from acid reflux. People with Barrett's esophagus are at increased risk for developing esophageal cancer. While there is no definitive answer to whether or not milk is safe to drink for people with Barrett's esophagus, some doctors recommend avoiding dairy products altogether. Milk is a common trigger for acid reflux, and it can also promote the growth of bacteria in the esophagus. For these reasons, it is best to err on the side of caution and avoid drinking milk if you have Barrett's esophagus. There are many other beverages that are safe to drink, including water, juices, and herbal teas. You may also want to avoid caffeine, alcohol, and carbonated beverages, as these can all trigger acid reflux. If you are not sure whether a particular beverage is safe for you to consume, talk to your doctor or a registered dietitian.

Does Vitamin D Help Barrett's esophagus?

Barrett's esophagus occurs when the lining of the esophagus is damaged, usually as a result of acid reflux. This can lead to a condition called GERD, or gastroesophageal reflux disease. GERD occurs when the stomach contents, including acid, flow back up into the esophagus. Over time, this can damage the esophageal lining and lead to Barrett's esophagus. There is some evidence that vitamin D may help to improve the symptoms of GERD and Barrett's esophagus. One study found that people with Barrett's esophagus who took vitamin D supplements had a lower risk of developing esophageal cancer. It's not clear exactly how vitamin D might help to improve the symptoms of Barrett's esophagus. One theory is that vitamin D helps to reduce inflammation in the digestive tract. Inflammation is thought to play a role in the development of Barrett's esophagus. Vitamin D is found in a variety of foods, including eggs, fortified milk, and fatty fish. You can also get vitamin D from exposure to sunlight. A simple blood test can determine if you are vitamin D deficient. If you have Barrett's esophagus, talk to your doctor about whether vitamin D supplements might be right for you.

Is Magnesium good for Barrett's esophagus?

Barrett's esophagus is a condition in which the tissues of the esophagus become damaged, usually as a result of acid reflux. Some experts believe that magnesium may help to protect the esophagus from damage caused by acid reflux. Magnesium is a mineral that is found in many foods, and it is also available in supplement form. Some studies have found that magnesium may help to reduce the symptoms of acid reflux, and it may also help to protect the esophagus from damage.

What vitamins are good for Barrett's esophagus?

Vitamins are an important part of a healthy diet. They can help your body function properly and keep you feeling your best. There are many different vitamins that are good for Barrett's esophagus, and you may need to take a supplement to get the right amounts. Talk to your doctor about what vitamins are best for you. Some vitamins that may be beneficial for Barrett's esophagus include vitamin C, vitamin D, and vitamin E. Vitamin C is an antioxidant that can help protect your cells from damage. It's also thought to boost your immune system. Vitamin D helps your body absorb calcium, which is important for strong bones and teeth. Vitamin E is an antioxidant that can help reduce inflammation. In addition to vitamins, there are other nutrients that can be beneficial for Barrett's esophagus. These include omega-3 fatty acids, magnesium, and probiotics. Omega-3 fatty acids are thought to have anti-inflammatory properties. They're found in fish, nuts, and seeds. Magnesium is a mineral that's important for many bodily functions. It can be found in green leafy vegetables, nuts, and seeds. Probiotics are live bacteria that are found in yogurt and other fermented foods. They're thought to have a variety of health benefits, including aiding in digestion. Eating a healthy diet is important for everyone, but it may be especially important if you have Barrett's esophagus. Talk to your doctor about what foods and nutrients you should include in your diet.

What is the death rate of Barrett's esophagus?

Barrett's esophagus is a condition in which the lining of the esophagus, the tube that carries food from the throat to the stomach, is replaced by tissue that is similar to the lining of the intestine. This condition is often associated with acid reflux, and it can increased a person's risk of esophageal cancer. The death rate of Barrett's esophagus is not well understood, as the condition is often diagnosed incidentally during an endoscopy for another reason. However, it is estimated that the risk of esophageal cancer in people with Barrett's esophagus is about 30-125 times higher than in the general population. While the overall risk of esophageal cancer is still low, it is important for people with Barrett's esophagus to be monitored closely by a doctor and to receive regular endoscopies.

The best way to avoid acid reflux is to change your diet. Avoiding fatty and spicy foods can help, as well as eating smaller meals and avoiding eating late at night. There are also over-the-counter and prescription medications that can help. If you have acid reflux, it is important to talk to your doctor to find the best treatment for you.

Is Barrett's esophagus a tumor?

Barrett's esophagus (BE) is a change in the lining of the esophagus that is associated with chronic gastroesophageal reflux disease (GERD). The condition is named after Norman Barrett, a British doctor who first described it in 1950. BE is considered a premalignant condition because people with BE are at an increased risk of developing esophageal adenocarcinoma (EAC), a type of cancer that forms in the tissues of the esophagus. While EAC is rare, it is one of the fastest-growing cancers in the United States and is often diagnosed at a late stage, when it is difficult to treat. The exact cause of BE is unknown, but it is thought to develop from repeated injury to the esophageal lining. This injury is thought to occur from the backflow of stomach acid and other digestive fluids into the esophagus (reflux). The main symptom of BE is heartburn, which is also a symptom of GERD. Other symptoms may include: • Chest pain • Difficulty swallowing • Regurgitation • Wheezing • Hoarseness A diagnosis of BE is made after an endoscopy, during which a small camera is passed through the mouth and into the esophagus. Biopsies (tissue samples) are taken during the endoscopy and examined under a microscope to look for changes in the cells of the esophagus. People with BE do not usually require treatment. However, they will need to be monitored closely because of the increased risk of developing EAC. Treatment for BE may be recommended if there are symptoms or if the biopsy results are abnormal. There are two main types of treatment for BE: medical and surgical. Medical treatment involves the use of medicines to decrease the amount of acid in the stomach. This can be done with antacids, H2 blockers, or proton pump inhibitors (PPIs). Surgical treatment involves removing a section of the esophagus with Barrett's and replacing it with healthy tissue. This is known as esophagectomy. Surgery is usually only recommended if medical treatment does not work or if there are abnormal biopsy results. BE is a condition that is associated with an increased risk of developing esophageal cancer. However, the majority of people with BE will never develop cancer. With proper monitoring and treatment, the risk of developing cancer can be greatly reduced.

Do you lose weight with Barrett's esophagus?

Barrett's esophagus is a condition in which the lining of the esophagus changes, becoming more like the lining of the intestine. This change is often a result of damage from acid reflux. While Barrett's esophagus can occur in people of any weight, it is more common in people who are overweight or obese. This may be because excess weight can contribute to acid reflux. One study found that people with Barrett's esophagus were more likely to be obese than people without the condition. The study also found that people with Barrett's esophagus were more likely to have a higher body mass index (BMI). While it is not clear if losing weight can reverse Barrett's esophagus, it may help to prevent the condition from getting worse. Losing weight can also help to reduce the symptoms of acid reflux. If you are overweight or obese, talk to your doctor about a weight loss plan that is right for you. Making lifestyle changes, such as eating a healthy diet and getting regular exercise, can help you lose weight and reduce your risk of Barrett's esophagus.

How do you get Barrett's esophagus?

Barrett's esophagus is a condition in which the lining of the esophagus is replaced by tissue that is similar to the lining of the intestine. This condition can be caused by acid reflux, which is a condition in which the stomach contents are regurgitated into the esophagus. Acid reflux can be caused by a variety of factors, such as overeating, eating spicy or fatty foods, drinking caffeine or alcohol, smoking, and pregnancy.

Can omeprazole reverse Barrett's esophagus?

Barrett's esophagus occurs when the lining of the esophagus is damaged, usually by acid reflux. This can lead to changes in the cells of the esophagus, which can eventually lead to cancer. Omeprazole is a medication that is used to treat acid reflux. It works by reducing the amount of acid that is produced by the stomach. Some studies have shown that omeprazole may be effective in reversing Barrett's esophagus. In one study, omeprazole was shown to reduce the severity of Barrett's esophagus and even reverse the condition in some people. However, more research is needed to confirm these results. Omeprazole is generally considered to be safe. However, there are some side effects that can occur, such as headaches, diarrhea, and nausea. If you are considering taking omeprazole for Barrett's esophagus, it is important to talk to your doctor first to make sure that it is the right medication for you.

How do you know if you have Barrett's Oesophagus?

Barrett's oesophagus is a condition in which the lining of the oesophagus, the tube that carries food from the mouth to the stomach, is replaced by a different type of tissue. This tissue is called columnar epithelium. Columnar epithelium is normally found in the intestine, but in Barrett's oesophagus, it is found in the oesophagus. This change is thought to be caused by damage to the oesophageal lining, possibly from stomach acid. Barrett's oesophagus is a serious condition because it can increase your risk of developing oesophageal cancer. Oesophageal cancer is a cancer that starts in the oesophagus. Most people with Barrett's oesophagus do not have any symptoms. The condition is often found during an investigation for another condition, such as gastro-oesophageal reflux disease (GORD). If you do have symptoms, they may include: • heartburn • trouble swallowing • chest pain • choking • feebleness • weight loss It's important to see your doctor if you have any of these symptoms. They may be caused by other conditions, such as GORD, so it's important to get a diagnosis. Your doctor will usually diagnose Barrett's oesophagus using an endoscopy. This is a procedure where a thin, flexible tube with a camera is passed down your throat so that your doctor can see your oesophagus. If Barrett's oesophagus is diagnosed, you'll be referred to a specialist for further treatment. This may involve having regular check-ups and surveillance endoscopies to check for signs of pre-cancerous changes in the tissue. In some cases, treatment to remove the abnormal tissue may be recommended.

As many as 60% of the adult population in the United States experiences acid reflux, also known as heartburn, at least once a year, and 20-30% suffer from it weekly. Despite its prevalence, there are many misconceptions about acid reflux. This article has addressed some of the most common myths about acid reflux, including that it is caused by stress, spicy food, and drinking alcohol. The truth is that acid reflux is caused by a weakening of the lower esophageal sphincter, which allows stomach acid to escape back up into the esophagus. While stress, spicy food, and alcohol can trigger symptoms, they are not the root cause of the condition. If you suffer from acid reflux, be sure to talk to your doctor about treatment options to help you find relief.

Occasional acid reflux

Acid reflux occurs when the sphincter at the bottom of the esophagus relaxes, allowing stomach acid to come up. This can happen due to a variety of reasons, including eating certain foods, lying down after eating, or wearing tight clothing. Acid reflux is usually not a serious problem, but it can be uncomfortable. There are a few things you can do to help reduce acid reflux. Avoiding trigger foods, eating smaller meals, and avoiding eating before lying down can all help. Additionally, over-the-counter medications like antacids can also be helpful in reducing symptoms. If you experience acid reflux regularly, you should talk to your doctor to see if there is a more serious underlying problem.

Silent reflux / Laryngopharyngeal Reflux (LPR)

Laryngopharyngeal reflux (LPR) is a condition in which acid and other stomach contents back up into the throat (pharynx). LPR can cause a silent cough and throat clearing, as well as a feeling of globus (a lump in the throat). Many people with LPR do not have heartburn, making it difficult to diagnose. LPR is caused by a weakened sphincter (the valve between the stomach and esophagus) that allows stomach contents to flow back up into the throat. This can happen when the stomach is overly full, or when lying down or bending over after eating. LPR is more than just heartburn. The symptoms of LPR can be divided into three categories: throat symptoms, airway symptoms, and extraesophageal (outside of the esophagus) symptoms. Throat symptoms: - A Lump in the Throat (Globus): The sensation that there is something stuck in the throat. This is caused by the inflammation of the esophagus and is often worse in the morning. - Throat Clearing: A constant need to clear the throat, which can be caused by postnasal drip, allergies, or Acid Reflux. - Hoarseness: A change in the quality of the voice, often described as sounding "raspy." This is caused by the inflammation of the vocal cords. Airway symptoms: - Coughing: A cough that is not due to a cold or other respiratory infection. This is the body's way of trying to remove the stomach contents that have entered the lungs. - Wheezing: A whistling sound when breathing, caused by the inflammation of the airways. - Asthma: Asthma can be aggravated by LPR, as the stomach contents that are breathed in can trigger an asthma attack. Extraesophageal symptoms: - Ear Pain: The stomach contents can irritate the eustachian tube, which connects the throat to the middle ear, causing ear pain. - Dental Erosion: The stomach acid can wear away the enamel on the teeth. LPR is diagnosed through a combination of a medical history, physical examination, and tests such as an upper GI series (x-ray of the esophagus, stomach, and upper intestine), endoscopy (a camera down the throat), pH monitoring (a test to measure the acidity in the esophagus), and impedance monitoring (a test to measure the movement of liquids and gases in the esophagus). LPR is treated with a combination of medication and lifestyle changes. Medications used to treat LPR include proton pump inhibitors (PPIs), H2 blockers, and antacids. PPIs are the most effective type of medication for LPR, as they work

Gerd / Gastroesophageal Reflux

Acid reflux, also called gastroesophageal reflux, is a common digestive disorder in which stomach acid flows back up from the stomach into the esophagus. This can cause heartburn, chest pain, and regurgitation. Acid reflux is typically treated with lifestyle changes, such as avoiding foods that trigger acid reflux, eating smaller meals, and avoiding eating late at night. In some cases, medications, such as antacids, are also used to treat symptoms. Surgery may be an option for severe cases.

Reflux esophagitis

Reflux esophagitis is a condition in which the esophagus, the tube that carries food from the mouth to the stomach, is inflamed and irritated by stomach acid. The esophagus is lined with a layer of mucus that protects it from the acid in the stomach. If this mucus layer is damaged, the esophagus can become very painful. There are a number of reasons why the mucus layer can be damaged, but one of the most common is a condition called GERD, or gastroesophageal reflux disease. This is when stomach acid regularly flows back up into the esophagus, causing the mucus layer to become inflamed and irritated. There are a number of treatments for reflux esophagitis, but the most effective is usually a combination of lifestyle changes and medication. Lifestyle changes may include avoiding trigger foods and drinks, losing weight, and avoiding smoking. Medications can help to reduce the amount of acid in the stomach, or to strengthen the mucus layer so that it is less likely to be damaged. If reflux esophagitis is left untreated, it can lead to serious complications such as ulcers, bleeding, and even cancer of the esophagus. Therefore, it is important to see a doctor if you think you may have this condition.

Barrett's esophagus

Barrett's esophagus is a disorder in which the tissue lining the esophagus becomes damaged, usually as a result of acid reflux. Acid reflux is a condition in which the stomach contents, including acid, back up into the esophagus. Over time, the acid can erode the lining of the esophagus, causing Barrett's esophagus. Barrett's esophagus is a serious condition that can lead to cancer of the esophagus. However, with early diagnosis and treatment, the chances of developing cancer are low. Symptoms of Barrett's esophagus include heartburn, dysphagia (difficulty swallowing), and regurgitation. These symptoms are similar to those of acid reflux, and many people with Barrett's esophagus do not experience any symptoms. If you have symptoms of Barrett's esophagus, your doctor will likely perform an endoscopy. During this procedure, a lighted tube is inserted down your throat and into your esophagus. Your doctor will then take a biopsy, or sample, of the tissue lining your esophagus. The biopsy will be sent to a laboratory for analysis. If you are diagnosed with Barrett's esophagus, your doctor will likely recommend treatment with proton pump inhibitors (PPIs). PPIs are medications that reduce the production of acid in the stomach. By reducing the amount of acid in the stomach, PPIs can help to heal the lining of the esophagus and prevent further damage. In some cases, surgery may be necessary to treat Barrett's esophagus. Surgery is usually only recommended if you have developed cancer of the esophagus.

Precancer or cancer

There is evidence to suggest that acid reflux may be a precursor to cancer, or may even cause cancer. This is because acid reflux can damage the lining of the esophagus, which can lead to changes in the DNA of the cells. These changes can then lead to cancer. Acid reflux is a condition in which stomach acid flows back up into the esophagus, the tube that carries food from the mouth to the stomach. This can happen if the valve between the stomach and the esophagus, known as the lower esophageal sphincter, is not working properly. Dysplasia is an early form of cell change that may lead to cancer. When the cells of the esophagus are damaged by acid reflux, they may undergo dysplasia. In dysplasia, the cells look abnormal under a microscope, but they are not cancer. However, dysplasia can progress to cancer. If you have acid reflux, you should see a doctor. There are treatments that can help to prevent further damage to the esophagus and reduce the risk of cancer.

Who's at risk for Acid Reflux

Acid reflux is a chronic condition in which stomach acids leak back up into the esophagus, causing heartburn and other painful symptoms. The condition affects people of all ages, but is most common in adults over age 40. There are several risk factors for acid reflux, including: Obesity: Obesity is a major risk factor for acid reflux. Studies show that the more weight you gain, the greater your risk of developing the condition. Pregnancy: Pregnant women are at increased risk for acid reflux due to the pressure of the growing fetus on the stomach and lower esophageal sphincter. Smoking: Smoking cigarettes can increase your risk of acid reflux by relaxes the lower esophageal sphincter and damages the lining of the esophagus. Certain Medications: Common culprits include antidepressants, antihistamines, and painkillers. Diet: Foods that are spicy, fatty, or acidic can trigger acid reflux. Eating large meals or lying down immediately after eating can also lead to heartburn. If you're experiencing heartburn or other symptoms of acid reflux more than twice a week, you may have acid reflux disease. Acid reflux disease is a serious condition that can lead to ulcers, Barrett's esophagus (a precancerous condition), and even cancer of the esophagus. If you think you may have acid reflux disease, talk to your doctor.

There are many possible causes of acid reflux, including diet, lifestyle, and medical conditions. Treatment focuses on reducing the production of stomach acid and easing symptoms. Some lifestyle changes that may help include avoiding trigger foods, eating smaller meals, and avoiding eating late at night. Medications that reduce stomach acid production or help move food through the stomach more quickly can also be effective. In some cases, surgery may be necessary.

What tea is good for acid reflux?

Acid reflux, also known as GERD, is a condition in which stomach acid flows back up into the esophagus, causing a burning sensation in the chest or throat. While there are a variety of over-the-counter and prescription medications available to treat acid reflux, many people find relief with natural remedies. One potential natural remedy for acid reflux is tea. Tea is thought to have several health benefits, including aiding in digestion and reducing inflammation. However, it's important to choose the right type of tea to drink if you're suffering from acid reflux. Some of the best teas for acid reflux include: -Ginger tea: Ginger has long been used as a natural remedy for indigestion and other stomach ailments. It can help to soothe the stomach and reduce acidity. - Chamomile tea: Chamomile is a type of herbal tea that is thought to be very helpful in relieving digestive issues. It is also thought to be a natural relaxant, which can help to reduce stress levels and promote a good night's sleep. - Green tea: Green tea is a type of tea that is rich in antioxidants and has been shown to have numerous health benefits. It's thought to be helpful in reducing inflammation and promoting digestion. All of these teas can be helpful in relieving symptoms of acid reflux. However, it's important to listen to your body and see what works best for you. If you find that a certain tea aggravates your symptoms, it's best to avoid it. In general, it's a good idea to avoid caffeine and acidic beverages if you're suffering from acid reflux. Instead, opt for soothing herbal teas that can help to reduce stomach acid and promote digestion.

* 9 7 8 1 7 7 6 9 6 9 8 4 5 *
SD - #0051 - 121026 - C0 - 229/152/13 - PB - 9781776969845 - Matt Lamination